Orthopedic and Athletic Injury Evaluation Handbook

Orthopedic and Athletic Injury Evaluation Handbook

Chad Starkey, PHD, ATC

Associate Professor
Bouvé College of Health Sciences
School of Health Professions
Boston, Massachusetts

Jeffrey L. Ryan, PT, ATC

Clinical Director
Hahnemann Sports Medicine Center
Hahnemann University Hospital
Philadelphia, Pennsylvania

 F. A. DAVIS COMPANY · PHILADELPHIA

F. A. Davis Company
1915 Arch Street
Philadelphia, PA 19103
www.fadavis.com

Copyright © 2003 by F. A. Davis Company

Printed in Canada

Last digit indicates print number: 10 9 8 7 6 5 4 3

Acquisitions Editor: Christa A. Fratantoro
Developmental Editor: Melissa A. Reed
Cover Designer: Louis J. Forgione

As new scientific information becomes available through basic and clinical research, recommended treatments and drug therapies undergo changes. The author(s) and publisher have done everything possible to make this book accurate, up to date, and in accord with accepted standards at the time of publication. The author(s), editors, and publisher are not responsible for errors or omissions or for consequences from application of the book, and make no warranty, expressed or implied, in regard to the contents of the book. Any practice described in this book should be applied by the reader in accordance with professional standards of care used in regard to the unique circumstances that may apply in each situation. The reader is advised always to check product information (package inserts) for changes and new information regarding dose and contraindications before administering any drug. Caution is especially urged when using new or infrequently ordered drugs.

Library of Congress Cataloging-in-Publication Data

Starkey, Chad, 1959-
  Evaluation of orthopedic and athletic injury handbook/Chad Starkey, Jeff Ryan
    p. ; cm.
  "Companion guide to the second edition of Evaluation of orthopedic and athletic injuries"-Pref.
  Includes bibliographical references and index.
  ISBN 0-8036-1104-8
    1. Sports injuries-Handbooks, manuals, etc. 2. Orthopedics-Handbooks, manuals, etc. I. Ryan, Jeffrey L., 1962- II. Starkey, Chad, 1959-. Evaluation of orthopedic and athletic injuries. III. Title.
    [DNLM: 1. Athletic Injuries-diagnosis-Handbooks. 2. Orthopedic Procedures-methods-Handbooks. QT 29 S795e 2003]
  RD97.S833 2003
  617.1'027-dc21.

2003043403

Imagination is a powerful deceiver.
—CAS

To my family, friends, and colleagues. Someone once said that success is doing what you love. One of my greatest successes in life is being associated with all of you.
—JLR

To Jean-François Vilain, thanks for your guidance, patience, and loyalty. Most of all, thanks for your friendship.
—CAS
JLR

Preface

The *Orthopedic and Athletic Injury Evaluation Handbook* was created for two purposes. First, it is a companion guide to *Evaluation of Orthopedic and Athletic Injuries*. It provides students and instructors an easy-to-carry, quick reference guide for use during laboratories and clinical affiliations. Second, it can also serve as a clinical reference guide and resource for practicing professionals. The *Handbook*, like other pocket guides commonly used in medicine, was designed for quick reference when access to the full textbook is not practical.

This text presents an overview of the relevant knowledge and skills required to perform a comprehensive clinical orthopedic and athletic injury examination. Although the *Handbook* includes information relevant to athletic injuries, it is appropriate for most orthopedic injury evaluations.

We have attempted to follow the flow and sequence of *Evaluation of Orthopedic and Athletic Injuries* as closely as possible. Chapter and Component tabs along the top and side margins should provide easy access to the information.

Each chapter begins with an evaluation "map" that describes the key components of the part of the body being evaluated. Relevant findings of the history and inspection phases are followed by key landmarks to be used during bony and soft-tissue palpation. Ultimately, the strength of the *Handbook* lies in the presentation of the range-of-motion, ligamentous, and special tests for the body parts. These sections provide detailed instructions on how to perform these tests, common modifications, and the implications of positive findings. When applicable, neurological examination is included in the chapter.

Nonorthopedic chapters include Head Injuries, Heat Illness, Cardio-respiratory, and Skin Conditions. The Handbook concludes with useful appendices describing upper and lower extremity reflex tests, assessment of muscle length, and lower extremity functional tests.

We would like to thank the staff at FA Davis, especially Susan Rhyner, Manager of Creative Development; Margaret Biblis, Publisher of Health Professions/Medicine; Ona Kosmos, Editorial Associate; and Melissa Reed, our Developmental Editor. Without their efforts in developing the text, this Handbook would not have been possible. We must also thank Christa Fratantoro, who made up for her lack of joke-telling acumen by first conceptualizing this Handbook. We had a whale of a time.

The following individuals have added their expertise through their careful reviews:

William Holcomb, PhD, ATC
Athletic Training Program Director
University of Nevada, Las Vegas
Las Vegas, NV

Peg Houglum, PhD, ATC, PT
Athletic Training Department
Assistant Professor
Duquesne University
Pittsburgh, PA

Peter B. Koehnke, MS, ATC
Sports Medicine
Professor and Chair
Canisius College
Buffalo, NY

Dan Sedory, MS, ATC
Department of Kinesiology
Curriculum Director, Assistant Professor
University of New Hampshire
Durham, NH

Contents

The Injury Evaluation Process

History
Determine the mechanism of injury and onset of the symptoms, and question the patient about any associated sounds or sensations at the time of injury. Ascertain any relevant history of prior injury to the involved and uninvolved sides. The history continues throughout the evaluation based on subsequent findings.

Inspection
Compare the involved and uninvolved sides for signs of swelling, deformity, differences in skin color and texture, muscle tone, and other bilateral differences. The inspection process begins during, or prior to, history taking and continues throughout the evaluation.

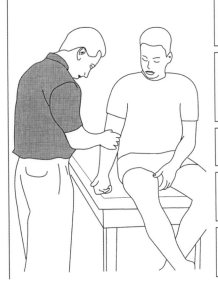

Palpation
Identify areas of point tenderness, crepitus, swelling, malalignment of a joint or bone, or other types of deformity.

Range of Motion Tests
Determine a joint's ability to move activety and passively through a range of motion and the joint's muscles ability to generate tension through resisted range of motion or manual muscle tests.

Ligamentous Tests
Apply a stress in one of the cardinal planes to a joint's ligaments and/or capsule.

Special Tests
Apply a stress (often in multiple planes) to isolate a specific anatomical structure or function.

Neurological Tests
Assess motor and sensory nerve function. Identify normal reflex loops. Not required for all evaluations.

2   CHAPTER 1   The Injury Evaluation Process

History

Table 1–1 Classification System for Overuse Injuries

Stage	Presentation of Symptoms	Functional Ability
I	Pain after activity	Little dysfunction initially; pain with movement increasing as the patient nears stage II
II	Pain during and after activity	Pain with movement of the body part, with associated decreased performance; in the latter stages, dysfunction of the body part may make the patient unable to perform activity
III	Constant pain	Great loss of function during all activities

Table 1–2 Conditions Warranting Termination of the Evaluation

Segment	Findings to Warrant Immediate Physician Referral
History	Reports of the inability to feel or move one or more limbs (confirm with neurological screen) Reports of significant chest pain Description of a general medical condition that could affect the outcome of the evaluation Reports of difficulty breathing (e.g., anaphylaxis)
Inspection	Obvious fracture Obvious joint dislocation
Palpation	Disruption in the contour of bone, indicating a fracture or joint dislocation Gross joint instability Malalignment of joint structures
Range of motion testing	Third-degree muscle tears
Ligamentous testing	Gross joint instability
Special tests	Gross joint instability
Neurological tests	Neurologic dysfunction Sensory dysfunction Motor dysfunction Absent or diminished reflexes

Inspection

Box 1–1   Girth Measurement

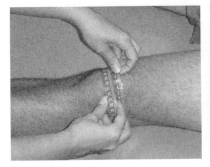 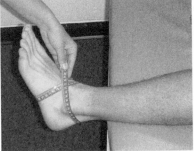

POSITION OF THE PATIENT	Supine
EVALUATIVE PROCEDURE	1. To determine capsular swelling, identify the joint line using prominent bony landmarks. To determine muscular atrophy, make incremental marks (e.g., 2, 4, and 6 in) from the joint line.
	2. Do not use a measuring tape made of cloth (cloth tapes tend to stretch and cause the markings to fade).
	3. Lay the measuring tape symmetrically around the body part, being careful not to fold or twist the tape. Use a figure-8 technique to measure ankle girth. Position the tape across the malleoli proximally and around the navicular and the base of the fifth metatarsal distally.
	3. Pull the tape snugly and read the circumference in centimeters or inches.
	4. Take three measurements and record the average.
	5. Repeat these steps for the uninjured limb.
	6. Record the findings in the medical file.
POSITIVE RESULTS	A significant difference in the girth between the two limbs, based on factors such as lower or upper extremity, side dominance, and so on.
IMPLICATIONS	Increased girth across the joint line: swelling Increased girth of muscle mass: hypertrophy Decreased girth of muscle mass: atrophy

Passive Range of Motion

Table 1–3 Physiological (Normal) End-Feels

End-Feel	Structure	Example
Soft	Soft tissue approximation	Knee flexion (contact between soft tissue of the posterior leg and posterior thigh)
Firm	Muscular stretch	Hip flexion with the knee extended (passive elastic tension of hamstring muscles)
	Capsular stretch	Extension of the metacarpophalangeal joints of the fingers (tension in the palmar capsule)
	Ligamentous stretch	Forearm supination (tension in the palmar radioulnar ligament of the inferior radioulnar joint, interosseous membrane, oblique cord)
Hard	Bone contacting bone	Elbow extension (contact between the olecranon process of the ulna and the olecranon fossa of the humerus)

Table 1–4 Pathological (Abnormal) End-Feels

End-Feel	Description	Example
Soft	Occurs sooner or later in the ROM than is usual or occurs in a joint that normally has a firm or hard end-feel; feels boggy	Soft tissue edema Synovitis
Firm	Occurs sooner or later in the ROM than is usual or occurs in a joint that normally has a soft or hard end-feel	Increased muscular tonus Capsular, muscular, ligamentous shortening
Hard	Occurs sooner or later in the ROM than is usual or occurs in a joint that normally has a soft or firm end-feel; feels like a bony block	Osteoarthritis Loose bodies in joint Myositis ossificans Fracture
Empty	Has no real end-feel because end of ROM is never reached owing to pain; no resistance felt except for patient's protective muscle splinting or muscle spasm	Acute joint inflammation Bursitis Abscess Fracture Psychogenic origin

Box 1–2 Goniometric Evaluation

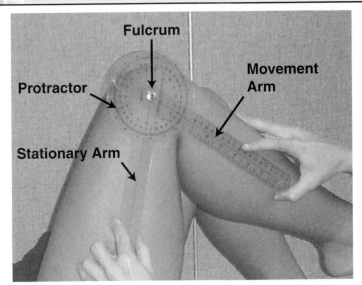

GONIOMETER SEGMENTS	PROTRACTOR:	Measures the arc of motion in degrees. Full-circle goniometers have a 360° protractor; half-circle goniometers have a 180° protractor.
	FULCRUM:	The center of the goniometer's axis of rotation
	STATIONARY ARM:	The portion of the goniometer that extends from, and is part of, the protractor
	MOVEMENT ARM:	The portion of the goniometer that moves independently from the protractor around an arc formed by the fulcrum

PROCEDURE

1. Select a goniometer of the appropriate size and shape for the joint being tested.
2. Position the joint in its starting position.
3. Identify the center of the joint's axis of motion.
4. Locate the proximal and distal landmarks along the long axis of the joint motion being tested.
5. Align the goniometer's fulcrum over the joint axis.
6. Align the stationary arm along the proximal body segment and the movement arm along the distal segment.
7. Read and record the starting values from the goniometer.
8. Move the distal joint segment through its range of motion.
9. Reapply the goniometer as described in Steps 5 and 6.
10. Read and record the ending values from the goniometer.

Resisted Range of Motion

Principles of Resisted Range of Motion Testing

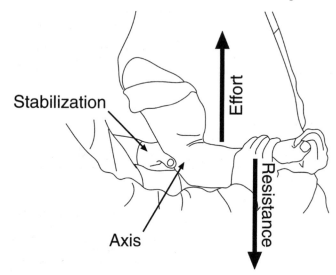

FIGURE 1–1 Performing manual resistance tests. The extremity is stabilized proximal to the joint being tested while resistance is provided distal to the joint.

Table 1–5 Grading Systems for Manual Muscle Tests		
Verbal	Numerical	Clinical Finding
Normal	5/5	The patient can resist against maximal pressure; the examiner is unable to break the patient's resistance.
Good	4/5	The patient can resist against moderate pressure.
Fair	3/5	The patient can move the body part against gravity through the full range of motion.
Poor	2/5	The patient can move the body part in a gravity-eliminated position through the full range of motion.
Trace	1/5	The patient cannot produce movement, but a muscle contraction is palpable.
Gone	0/5	No contraction is felt.

Table 1–6 Findings in Resisted Range of Motion Tests

Strength	Pain	Clinical Indication
Good	None	Normal
Good	Present	Minor contractile soft tissue injury
Weak	Present	Significant contractile soft tissue injury
Weak	None	Neurological deficit or chronic contractile soft tissue injury

Ligamentous Tests

Table 1–7 Grading System for Ligamentous Laxity

Grade	Ligamentous End-Feel	Damage
I	Firm (normal)	Slight stretching of the ligament with little, if any, tearing of the fibers. Pain is present, but the degree of laxity roughly compares with that of the opposite extremity.
II	Soft	Partial tearing of the fibers. There is increased glide of the joint surfaces upon one another or the joint line "opens up" significantly when compared with the opposite side.
III	Empty	Complete tearing of the ligament. The motion is excessive and becomes restricted by other joint structures, such as secondary restraints or tendons.

Process

Neurological Tests

Dermatomes

View of Dorsal Surface

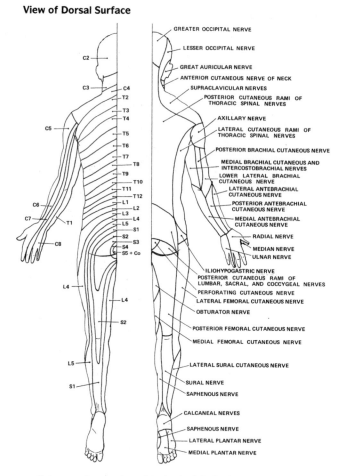

Cutaneous innervation of the back of the body. Dermatomes are on the left, and peripheral nerves are on the right.

FIGURE 1–2 The body's dermatomes. These charts describe the area of skin receiving sensory input from each of the nerve roots. Note that there are many different dermatome references, thus explaining the inconsistencies from text to text.

Neurological Tests

Dermatomes

View of Ventral Surface

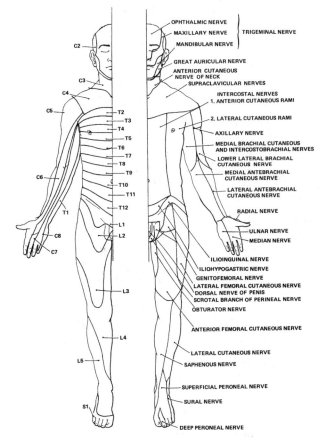

Cutaneous innervation of the front of the body. Dermatomes are on the left, and peripheral nerves are on the right.

FIGURE 1-2 (Continued).

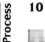

Process

BILATERAL

Box 1–3 Lower Quarter Neurological Screen

Dermatome

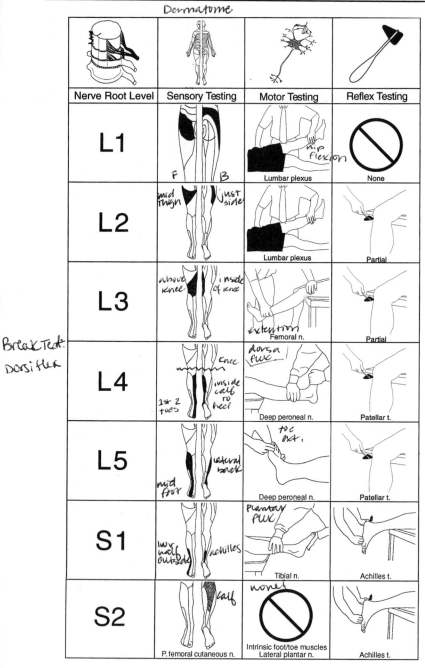

Break Test:
Dorsiflex

Nerve Root Level	Sensory Testing	Motor Testing	Reflex Testing
L1	F B	hip flexion	None
		Lumbar plexus	
L2	mid thigh / just side		Partial
		Lumbar plexus	
L3	above knee / inside of knee	extension / Femoral n.	Partial
L4	knee / inside calf to heel / 1st 2 toes	dorsa flex / Deep peroneal n.	Patellar t.
L5	lateral back / mid foot	toe ext. / Deep peroneal n.	Patellar t.
S1	lwr calf outside / achilles	plantar flex / Tibial n.	Achilles t.
S2	calf / P. femoral cutaneous n.	none / Intrinsic foot/toe muscles Lateral plantar n.	Achilles t.

Box 1–4 Upper Quarter Neurological Screen

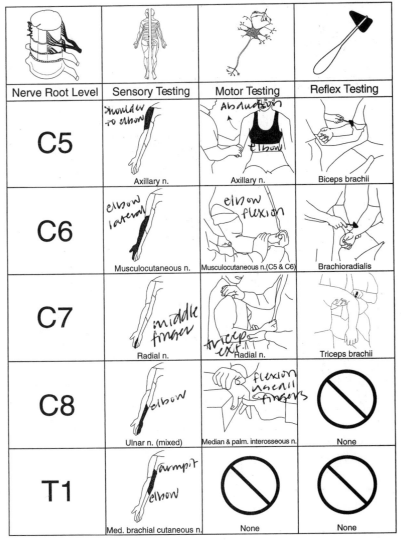

Nerve Root Level	Sensory Testing	Motor Testing	Reflex Testing
C5	shoulder to elbow / Axillary n.	Abduction elbow / Axillary n.	Biceps brachii
C6	elbow lateral / Musculocutaneous n.	elbow flexion / Musculocutaneous n.(C5 & C6)	Brachioradialis
C7	middle finger / Radial n.	triceps ext / Radial n.	Triceps brachii
C8	elbow / Ulnar n. (mixed)	flexion uncail fingers / Median & palm. interosseous n.	None
T1	armpit elbow / Med. brachial cutaneous n.	None	None

Brachial Plexus

nerve passes above the bone

2

Injury Nomenclature

Strains

- **First-degree strains** involve stretching of the muscle fibers. Pain increases as the muscle contracts, especially against resistance, and the site of injury is point tender. Swelling may also be present.
- **Second-degree strains** involve the actual tearing of some of the muscle fibers and may cause ecchymosis. These injuries present with the same findings as first-degree strains but are more severe.
- **Third-degree strains** involve the complete rupture of the muscle, resulting in a total loss of function and a palpable defect in the muscle. Pain, swelling, and ecchymosis are also present.

Sprains

- **First-degree sprain:** The ligament is stretched with little or no tearing of its fibers. No abnormal motion is produced when the joint is stressed, and a firm *end-point* is felt. Local pain, mild point tenderness, and slight swelling of the joint are present.
- **Second-degree sprain:** Partial tearing of the ligament's fibers has occurred, resulting in joint laxity when the ligament is stressed. A soft but definite end-point is present. Moderate pain and swelling occur, and a loss of the joint's function is noted.
- **Third-degree sprain:** The ligament has been completely ruptured, causing gross joint laxity, possible instability, and an empty or absent end-point. Swelling is marked, but pain may be limited secondary to tearing of the local nerves. A complete loss of function of the joint is usually noted.

Tendinitis

- **First-degree tendinitis** is marked by pain and slight dysfunction during activity.

- **Second-degree tendinitis** results in decreased function and pain after activity.
- **Third-degree tendinitis** is characterized by constant pain that prohibits activity.

Soft Tissue Injuries

Table 2–1 EVALUATIVE FINDINGS: Muscle Strains

Examination Segment	Clinical Findings	
History	*Onset:*	Acute. Pain is located at the site of the injury, which tends to be at or near the junction between the muscle belly and tendon. The distal musculotendinous junction is most often involved.
	Pain characteristics:	Pain is located at the site of the injury, which tends to be at or near the junction between the muscle belly and tendon.
	Mechanism:	Strains usually result from a single episode of overstretching or overloading of the muscle but are more likely to result from eccentric loading.
	Predisposing conditions:	Muscle tightness and improper warm-up before activity may predispose individuals to strain.
Inspection	Ecchymosis is evident in cases of severe muscle strains. Gravity causes the blood to pool distal to the site of trauma. Swelling may be present over the involved area. In severe cases, a defect may be visible in the muscle or tendon. If the strain involves a muscle of the lower extremity, the patient may walk with a limp.	
Palpation	Point tenderness exists over the site of the injury, with the degree of pain increasing with the severity of the injury. A defect or spasm may be palpable at the injury site.	
Range of motion	*AROM:*	Pain is elicited at the injury site. In the case of second- or third-degree strains, the patient may be unable to complete the movement.
	PROM:	Pain is elicited at the injury site during passive motion in the direction opposite that of the muscle, placing it on stretch.
	RROM:	Muscle strength is reduced. Pain increases as the amount of resistance is increased. Third-degree strains result in a total loss of function.

AROM = active range of motion; PROM = passive range of motion; RROM = resisted range of motion.

Injury Nomenclature

Table 2-2 EVALUATIVE FINDINGS: Tendinitis

Examination Segment	Clinical Findings	
History	*Onset:*	Occurs gradually or is chronic
	Pain characteristics:	Pain exists throughout the tendon.
	Mechanism:	Results from microtraumatic forces applied to the tendon
	Predisposing conditions:	History of muscle tightness, poor conditioning, increase in the frequency, duration, and/or intensity of training, changes in footwear or surfaces
Inspection	Swelling may be noted. If the inflammation involves a tendon of the lower extremity, the patient may walk with a limp or demonstrate some other compensatory gait. Inflammation involving the upper extremity results in abnormal movement patterns. Many tendons are not directly visible or palpable.	
Palpation	The tendon is tender to the touch. Crepitus or thickening of the tendon may be noted.	
Range of motion	*AROM:*	Pain in the tendon is possible throughout the range of motion as force is generated within the tendon.
	PROM:	Pain is elicited during the extremes of the range of motion as the tendon is stretched. Pain can be elicited earlier in the ROM in more severe cases.
	RROM:	Strength is decreased by pain. Pain is increased when the joint is isometrically stressed in its non–weight-bearing position.

AROM = active range of motion; PROM = passive range of motion; RROM = resisted range of motion.

Table 2-3 EVALUATIVE FINDINGS: Myositis Ossificans

Examination Segment	Clinical Findings	
History	*Onset:*	The initial trauma is a hematoma caused by a single acute or repeated blows to the muscle. The ossification occurs gradually.
	Pain characteristics:	Pain occurs at the site of ossification, usually the site of a large muscle mass that is exposed to blows (e.g. the quadriceps femoris or biceps brachii muscles).
	Mechanism:	Calcium within the muscle fascia secondary to an abnormality in the healing process.
Palpation	Acutely, the muscle is tender. As the ossification develops, it may become palpable within the muscle mass. Swelling and warmth may be felt at the site of injury. A fever may develop.	
Range of motion	*AROM:*	As the ossification grows, the number of contractile units available to the muscle decreases. Antagonist motion is painful secondary to decreased flexibility within the affected muscle mass.
	PROM:	Decreased secondary to pain and adhesions within the muscle
	RROM:	Decreased secondary to pain; the ossification does not allow the muscle to contract normally
Special tests	Radiographic examination shows the ossification as it matures. A bone scan may be positive in the earlier stages.	

AROM = active range of motion; PROM =passive range of motion; RROM = resisted range of motion.

Injury Nomenclature

Table 2–4   EVALUATIVE FINDINGS: Bursitis

Examination Segment	Clinical Findings	
History	Onset:	Acute in the case of direct trauma to the bursa; insidious in the case of overuse or infection.
	Pain characteristics:	Pain occurring at the site of the bursal sac.
	Mechanism:	**Chemical:** Calcium or other chemical deposits within the bursa activating the inflammatory response. **Mechanical:** Repetitive rubbing of the soft tissue over a bony prominence or a direct blow, possibly related to improper biomechanics. **Septic:** Viral or bacterial invasion of the bursa.
	Predisposing conditions:	Improper biomechanics, poor padding of at-risk bursae (e.g., suprapatellar bursa, olecranon bursa).
Inspection	Local swelling of bursae can be very pronounced, especially those located over the olecranon process and patella. Chronic or septic bursitis may appear red.	
Palpation	Point tenderness is noted over the site of the bursa. Localized heat and swelling may be noted.	
Range of motion	AROM:	Pain may be noted.
	PROM:	Pain is produced if the motion causes the tendon or other structure to rub across the inflamed bursa.
	RROM:	Pain limits RROM. As the muscle contracts, it compresses the bursal sac.

AROM = active range of motion; PROM = passive range of motion; RROM = resisted range of motion.

Table 2–5 EVALUATIVE FINDINGS: Ligament Sprains

Examination Segment	Clinical Findings	
History	*Onset:*	Acute
	Pain characteristics:	Pain is localized to the site of injury with first-degree sprains. As the severity of the sprain increases, the pain is radiated throughout the joint. A "popping" sensation or sound may be reported by the patient.
	Mechanism:	Sprains result from tensile forces caused by the stretching of the ligament.
	Predisposing conditions:	A history of a sprain can predispose the ligament to further injury. Shoe wear that increases the friction between the shoe–surface interface may increase the chance of lower extremity sprains. Women have a greater risk of some knee ligament sprains, but the exact cause has not been determined.
Inspection	Swelling of the joint is evident. Ecchymosis may form at and distal to the site of injury.	
Palpation	Point tenderness is noted over the ligament. The entire joint may be tender.	
Functional tests	*AROM:*	Limited by pain in the direction that stresses the involved ligament (or ligaments)
	PROM:	Limited by pain, especially in the direction that stresses the involved ligament (or ligaments)
	RROM:	Manual resistance throughout the ROM is painful. Isometric contractions may not produce as intense pain.
Ligamentous tests	The ligament can be stressed by producing a force through the joint that causes the ligament to stretch. The examiner should note the amount of increased laxity compared with the opposite side, as well as the quality of the end-point. The end-point should be distinct and crisp. A soft, "mushy," or absent end-point is a sign of ligamentous rupture.	
Special tests	These are determined by the particular joint being examined.	

AROM = active range of motion; PROM = passive range of motion; ROM = range of motion; RROM = resisted range of motion.

Table 2–6 EVALUATIVE FINDINGS: Joint Subluxations

Examination Segment	Clinical Findings	
History	*Onset:*	Acute or chronic. Chronic subluxation can occur as the joint's supportive structures are progressively stretched.
	Pain characteristics:	Pain occurs throughout the involved joint. Associated muscle spasm may involve the muscles proximal and distal to the joint.
	Mechanism:	Joint subluxation results from a stress that takes the joint beyond its normal anatomical limits.
	Predisposing conditions:	History of joint subluxation; congenital hyperlaxity
Inspection	Swelling may be present. No gross bony deformity is noted because the joint relocates.	
Palpation	Pain elicited along the tissues that have been stretched or compressed.	
Functional tests	*AROM:*	Possibly limited owing to pain and possible instability.
	PROM:	Possibly limited owing to pain and possible instability.
	RROM:	Muscular strength is decreased secondary to pain and joint instability.
Ligamentous tests	Pain is elicited during stress testing of the involved ligament (or ligaments). Laxity of the tissues is present, particularly post-acutely. The patient may note instability and react to guard against this by contracting the surrounding musculature or pulling away, an apprehension response.	
Special tests	These vary according to the body part being tested.	

AROM = active range of motion; PROM = passive range of motion; RROM = resisted range of motion.

Table 2–7 EVALUATIVE FINDINGS: Joint Dislocations

Examination Segment	Clinical Findings	
History	Onset:	Acute or chronic. Chronic dislocation as the joint's supportive structures are progressively stretched
	Pain characteristics:	At the involved joint
	Mechanism:	Dislocation caused by a stress that forces the joint beyond its normal anatomical limits
Inspection	Gross joint deformity may be present and swelling is observed.	
Palpation	Pain is elicited throughout the joint. Malalignment of the joint surfaces may be felt.	
Functional tests	ROM is not possible because of the disruption of the joint's alignment.	
Ligamentous tests	These are contraindicated when the joint is dislocated.	
Special tests	Except for checking neurovascular injury, these are contraindicated when the joint is dislocated.	
Neurological tests	Sensory distribution distal to the dislocated joint must be established.	
Comments	Dislocations of the major joints represent medical emergencies. The presence of the distal pulse must be established. A lack of circulation to the distal extremity threatens the viability of the body part.	

ROM = range of motion.

Injury Nomenclature

Table 2–8 EVALUATIVE FINDINGS: Capsular Synovitis

Examination Segment	Clinical Findings	
History	Onset:	Insidious; often subsequent to a previous injury to the joint
	Pain characteristics:	Pain occurring throughout the entire joint, causing aching at rest and increased pain with activity
	Mechanism:	Synovitis often begins following an injury to a joint. The resulting inflammatory reaction triggers inflammation within the synovium.
	Predisposing conditions:	Underlying pathology within the joint
Inspection	The joint may appear swollen. The patient may move the joint in a guarded manner. Joints affected by synovitis do not appear red. Persistent synovitis can result in muscle atrophy secondary to pain and decreased joint ROM.	
Palpation	Warmth may be felt. A "boggy" swelling is present. No distinct area of point tenderness is usually present.	
Functional tests	AROM:	Limitations exist within the capsular pattern of the joint.
	PROM:	Normally, this is greater than AROM but is still limited by pain.
	RROM:	Weakness secondary to muscle guarding
Ligamentous tests	In the absence of underlying pathology to the ligaments, the ligamentous test result is negative. Pain may be elicited by stretching the inflamed tissues.	
Special tests	Same findings are produced as for ligamentous testing	
Comments	The signs and symptoms of synovitis may mimic those of an infected joint.	

AROM = active range of motion; PROM = passive range of motion; RROM = resisted range of motion.

Table 2–9 EVALUATIVE FINDINGS: Osteochondral Defects	
Examination Segment	**Clinical Findings**
History	*Onset:* Acute or insidious
	Pain characteristics: Complaints of pain in the joint during weight-bearing activities, depending on the site of the defect, the entire joint may be painful secondary to a synovial reaction (see Synovitis)
	Mechanism: Acute: A rotational or ***axial load*** placed on two opposing joint surfaces. The resulting friction results in a tearing away of the cartilage.
	Chronic: A progressive degeneration of the articular cartilage.
	Predisposing conditions: None
Inspection	Effusion is present.
Palpation	The joint line may be tender from the defect, but the defect itself is usually not palpable. Tenderness may also be caused by synovitis.
Functional tests	*AROM:* Limited owing to pain and swelling
	PROM: Increased relative to the AROM but still limited by pain and swelling
	RROM: Decreased strength occurs, secondary to pain.
Special tests	The defect may be present on standard radiographic examination. Better imaging is obtained through the use of MRI.

AROM = active range of motion; MRI = magnetic resonance imaging; PROM = passive range of motion; RROM = resisted range of motion.

Injury Nomenclature

Table 2-10	**EVALUATIVE FINDINGS: Osteochondritis Dissecans**	
Examination Segment	**Clinical Findings**	
History	*Onset:*	Insidious or acute
	Pain characteristics:	Pain occurring within the joint, increasing with motion and possibly absent when the joint is at rest
	Mechanism:	Insidious: Progressive degeneration of the joint structures. Acute: Trauma causing a piece of bone or cartilage to break free and enter the joint space.
Inspection	Swelling around the joint may be noted. The patient tends to hold the joint in a pain-free position.	
Palpation	The affected joint may feel warm secondary to inflammation. Pain may become specific on palpation along the joint line.	
Functional tests	AROM, PROM, and RROM may be reduced secondary to the loose body's lodging between the joint surfaces, creating a mechanical block against movement.	
	AROM:	May be limited by pain, contracture, or locking secondary to a loose body
	PROM:	May be limited by pain, contracture, or locking secondary to a loose body
	RROM:	May be limited by pain or contracture
Comments	Osteochondritis dissecans is categorized by the age of onset, juvenile (under age 15 years) and adult (age 15 years or older).	

AROM = active range of motion; PROM = passive range of motion; RROM = resisted range of motion.

Table 2–11 EVALUATIVE FINDINGS: Arthritis

Examination Segment	Clinical Findings	
History	*Onset:*	Insidious
	Pain characteristics:	Pain occurs throughout the involved joint.
	Mechanism:	Osteoarthritis develops secondary to trauma and irregular biomechanical stresses being placed across the joint. Rheumatoid arthritis is caused by a systemic disorder that activates an inflammatory response in the body's joints.
	Predisposing conditions:	For osteoarthritis, previous trauma to the joint has occurred. Rheumatoid arthritis is associated with a family history of the disorder. Certain occupations and obesity may overload the joints, causing increased forces over time.
Inspection	In chronic cases, gross deformity of the joint is noticed. Individuals with cases of shorter duration present with swelling. When arthritis affects the joints of the lower extremity, an antalgic gait is produced.	
Palpation	Warmth and swelling are identified in the affected joint. The articular surfaces, when and where palpable, are tender to the touch.	
Functional tests	*AROM:*	May be limited by pain, often becoming contractured as the condition progresses
	PROM:	These findings are equal to those of AROM testing.
	RROM:	This is decreased secondary to pain.
Ligamentous tests	Test results may be positive if a deformity has developed, causing the stressed capsule and ligaments to elongate over time.	
Special tests	Radiographic examination and other imaging techniques show degenerative changes within the joint.	

AROM = active range of motion; PROM = passive range of motion; RROM = resisted range of motion.

Injury Nomenclature

BONY INJURIES

Table 2–12 EVALUATIVE FINDINGS: Exostosis

Examination Segment	Clinical Findings	
History	Onset:	Insidious
	Pain characteristics:	Exostosis involving the extremities most often results in the localization of pain and other symptoms. Spinal exostosis can result in pain being referred along the distribution of affected nerve roots.
	Mechanism:	Exostosis is the result of repeated strain placed on a bone or the bony insertion of a tendon.
	Predisposing conditions:	Previous trauma to the area
Inspection	Deformity may be noted over the site of pain.	
Palpation	Point tenderness is present. A defect, in the form of a bony outgrowth, may be palpable.	
Functional tests	AROM:	Limited secondary to pain and/or bony block
	PROM:	Equal to AROM
	RROM:	Reduced secondary to pain and/or bony block

AROM = active range of motion; PROM = passive range of motion; RROM = resisted range of motion.

Table 2–13 EVALUATIVE FINDINGS: Stress Fractures

Examination Segment	Clinical Findings	
History	Onset:	Insidious; the patient cannot report a single traumatic event causing the pain
	Pain characteristics:	Pain tends to radiate from the involved bone but may become diffuse.
	Mechansim:	Cumulative microtrauma causes stress fractures.
	Predisposing conditions:	Overtraining, poor conditioning, and improper training techniques may be noted.

Table 2–13   EVALUATIVE FINDINGS: Stress Fractures (Continued)

Examination Segment	Clinical Findings
Inspection	Usually no bony abnormality is noted. Soft tissue swelling and redness may be present.
Palpation	Point tenderness exists over the fracture site.
Functional tests	All motions are generally within normal limits.
Special tests	Long bone compression test Percussion along the length of the bone Bone scans or other imaging techniques

Box 2–1   Terminology Used to Describe the Fracture Location

Diaphyseal fractures involve only the bone's diaphysis and are associated with a good prognosis for recovery, barring any extenuating circumstances.

Epiphyseal fractures involve the fracture line crossing the bone's unsealed epiphyseal line and can have long-term consequences by disrupting the bone's normal growth. Epiphyseal fractures may mimic soft tissue injuries by resembling joint laxity during stress testing.

Articular fractures disrupt the joint's articular cartilage, which, if improperly healed, results in pain and decreased range of motion and can lead to arthritis of the joint.

Box 2-2 Terminology Used to Describe the Relative Severity of the Fracture Line

Fracture lines not completely disassociating the proximal end of the bone from its distal end are described as **incomplete fractures.**

Fracture lines with complete disassociation between the two ends of the bone are termed **undisplaced fractures** if the two ends of the bone maintain their relative alignment to each other.

The loss of alignment between the two segments is termed a **displaced fracture** and may jeopardize the surrounding tissues.

When a displaced fracture exits the skin, an **open fracture** (compound fracture) occurs.

Box 2-3 Terminology Used to Describe the Shape of the Fracture Line

Depressed fractures occur from direct trauma to flat bones, causing the bone to fracture and depress.

Transverse fractures are caused by a direct blow, *shear force,* or tensile force being applied to the shaft of a long bone and result in a fracture line that crosses the bone's long axis.

A **comminuted fracture** can result from extremely high-velocity impact forces leading to the shattering of bone into multiple pieces. This type of fracture often requires surgical correction.

A **compacted fracture** results from compressive forces placed through the long axis of the bone. One end of a fractured segment is driven into the opposite piece of the fracture, often leading to a shortening of the involved limb.

A **spiral fracture** results from a rotational force placed on the shaft of a long bone, such as twisting the tibia while the foot remains fixated. The fracture line assumes an S-shape along the length of the bone.

Longitudinal fractures, which most commonly occur as the result of a fall, have a fracture line that runs parallel to the bone's long axis.

Greenstick fractures, generally specific to the pediatric and adolescent population, involve a displaced fracture on one side of the bone and a compacted fracture on the opposite side. The name is derived from an analogy to an immature tree branch that has been snapped.

3

Assessment of Posture

SHERI L. MARTIN, MPT, ATC

Box 3–1 Classifications of Body Types

	Ectomorph	**Mesomorph**	**Endomorph**
Description	Slender, thin build; relatively low body weight	Medium, athletic build; relatively average body weight	Short, stocky build; relatively high body weight
Joint shape	Small, flat joint surfaces	Medium joint surfaces	Large, concave-convex joint surfaces
Muscle mass	Minimal muscle bulk, thin muscles	Medium muscle build	Thick muscle mass
Joint mobility	Increased	Within normal limits	Decreased
Joint stability	Decreased	Within normal limits	Increased

28

Box 3-2 Assessment of Ideal Posture

Lateral

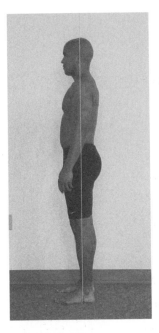

Alignment relative to plumb line:

Lower Extremity
- Lateral malleolus: Slightly posterior
- The tibia should be parallel to the plumb line and the foot should be at a 90° angle to the tibia
- Lateral femoral condyle: Slightly anterior
- Greater trochanter: Plumb line bisects

Torso
- Midthoracic region: Plumb line bisects

Shoulder
- Acromion process: Plumb line bisects

Head and Neck
- Cervical bodies: Plumb line bisects
- Auditory meatus: Plumb line bisects

Posture

Box 3–2 Assessment of Ideal Posture (Continued)

Anterior

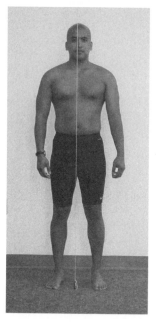

Alignment relative to plumb line:

Lower Extremity
- Feet: Evenly spaced from plumb line
- Tibial crests: Slight external rotation
- Knees: Evenly spaced from plumb line
- Patella: Facing anteriorly
- Consistent angulation from joint to joint
- The lateral malleoli, fibular head, and iliac crests should be bilaterally equal

Torso
- Umbilicus: Plumb line bisects
- Sternum: Plumb line bisects
- Jugular notch: Plumb line bisects

Shoulder
- Acromion processes: Evenly spaced from plumb line
- Shoulder heights equal or dominant side slightly lower
- Deltoid, anterior chest musculature bilaterally symmetrical and defined

Head and Neck
- Head is bisected by plumb line
- Nasal bridge: Plumb line bisects
- Frontal bone: Plumb line bisects

Box 3-2 Assessment of Ideal Posture (Continued)

Posterior

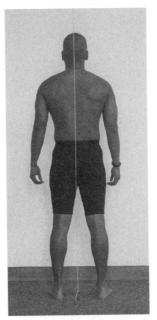

Alignment relative to plumb line:

Lower Extremity
- Feet evenly spaced from plumb line
- Feet in slight lateral rotation: Lateral 2 toes are visible
- Knees evenly spaced from plumb line
- Consistent angulation from joint to joint

Torso
- Median sacral crests: Plumb line bisects
- Spinous processes: Plumb line bisects
- Paraspinals bilaterally symmetrical

Shoulder
- Scapular borders: Evenly spaced from plumb line
- Acromion processes: Evenly spaced from plumb line
- Deltoid, posterior musculature bilaterally symmetrical
- Shoulder heights equal or dominant side slightly lower

Head and Neck
- Cervical spinous processes: Plumb line bisects
- Occipital protuberance: Plumb line bisects

Posture

Table 3–1   Postural Deviations Observed from the Lateral View

Body Region	Deviation from Ideal Posture	Structural Relationships
Talocrural joint	Dorsiflexion Plantarflexion	Knee flexion, hip flexion Genu recurvatum, knee extension, hip extension
Knee joint	Lateral epicondyle posterior to plumb line Lateral epicondyle anterior to plumb line	Knee hyperextension (genu recurvatum), ankle plantarflexion Knee flexion and ankle dorsiflexion
Hip joint	Greater trochanter posterior to plumb line Greater trochanter anterior to plumb line	Hip flexion, anterior pelvic tilt, increased lumbar lordosis Hip extension, posterior pelvic tilt, decreased lumbar lordosis
Pelvic position	Angle between ASIS and ipsilateral PSIS greater than 10°: Anterior pelvic tilt Angle between ASIS and ipsilateral PSIS less than 8°: Posterior pelvic tilt	Increased lumbar lordosis, hip flexion Decreased lumbar lordosis, hip extension
Lumbar spine	Lumbar vertebral bodies anterior to plumb line: Increased lumbar lordosis Lumbar vertebral bodies posterior to plumb line: Decreased lumbar lordosis	Anterior pelvic tilt, hip flexion Posterior pelvic tilt, hip extension
Thoracic spine	Midthorax posterior to plumb line: Increased thoracic kyphosis Midthorax anterior to plumb line: Decreased thoracic kyphosis	Forward head posture, forward shoulder posture, shortened anterior chest musculature Inability to flex through thoracic spine, possible shortened thoracic paraspinal muscles
Shoulder joint	Acromion process posterior to plumb line: Retracted shoulders or scapulae Acromion process anterior to plumb line: Rounded shoulder or protracted scapulae	Decreased thoracic kyphosis Forward head posture, increased thoracic kyphosis, shortened anterior chest musculature, poor postural control of the scapula
Cervical spine	Lower cervical vertebral bodies posterior to plumb line: Decreased cervical lordosis Lower cervical vertebral bodies anterior to plumb line: Increased cervical lordosis	Straightened cervical spine, muscle imbalances Forward head posture, forward shoulder posture, muscle imbalances
Head position	External auditory meatus posterior to plumb line: Head retraction External auditory meatus anterior to plumb line: Forward head posture	Straightened cervical spine, muscle imbalances Forward shoulder posture, muscle imbalances, suboccipital restrictions

ASIS = anterior superior iliac spine; PSIS = posterior superior iliac spine.

Table 3-2 Postural Deviations Observed from the Anterior View

Body Region	Deviation from Ideal Posture	Structural Relationships
Feet	Internally rotated feet (pigeon-toed)	Internal rotation of tibia, femoral anteversion, or STJ pronation
	Externally rotated feet (duck feet)	External rotation of tibia, femoral retroversion, or STJ supination
STJ	Flattened medial arch	Excessive STJ pronation, internal tibial rotation
	High medial arch	Excessive STJ supination, external tibial rotation
Tibial position	External tibial rotation: Tibial crests positioned lateral to midline	Femoral retroversion, STJ supination, lateral positioning of patella
	Internal tibial rotation: Tibial crests positioned medial to midline	Femoral anteversion, STJ pronation, medial positioning of patella
Patellar position	Squinting patellae	Internal tibial rotation, femoral anteversion, STJ pronation
	Frog-eyed patellae	External tibial rotation, femoral retroversion, STJ supination
Leg positions	Genu varum	Increased angle of inclination of femur, femoral retroversion, STJ supination
	Genu valgum	Decreased angle of inclination of femur, femoral anteversion, STJ pronation
	Tibial varum	Structural deformity of the tibias causing excessive STJ pronation
Pelvic position	The iliac crests asymmetrical	Leg length discrepancy, scoliosis
	The ASIS asymmetrical	One ilium is rotated either anteriorly or posteriorly, leg length discrepancy, or congenital anomaly
Chest region	Pectus carinatum: Outward protrusion of the chest and sternum	Structural anomaly
	Pectus excavatum: Inward position of the chest and sternum	Structural anomaly
Shoulder region	The shoulder heights asymmetrical	Scoliosis
Head and cervical spine	The head side bent or rotated; asymmetrical muscle mass of neck	Poor postural sense, overuse of one side, torticollis (congenital deformation or acute spasm of the sternocleidomastoid muscle)

ASIS = anterior superior iliac spine; STJ = subtalar joint.

Posture

Posture

Table 3–3	Postural Deviations Observed from the Posterior View	
Body Region	**Deviation from Ideal Posture**	**Structural Relationships**
Calcaneal position	Calcaneal varum Calcaneal valgum	STJ in a supinated position STJ in a pronated position
Posterior leg musculature	Asymmetry in girth or definition of musculature	Leg side dominance Atrophy caused by injury or immobilization of one side
Iliac crest heights	Asymmetry of iliac crest heights	Possible leg length discrepancy Scoliosis
Back musculature	Asymmetry between mass or definition of erector spinae musculature	Side dominance or overuse of one side of the musculature (e.g., crew) Scoliosis
Spinal alignment	The spinous processes not in vertical alignment	A structural or functional scoliosis Asymmetry of scapula Asymmetry of spinal musculature Asymmetry of rib cage
Scapular position	Unequal height	Side dominance Scoliosis Muscle imbalance caused by paralysis or weakness of musculature
	Excessively protracted or asymmetrically protracted	Muscle imbalance Poor posture Scoliosis Forward shoulder posture Forward head posture
	Asymmetrically rotated	Muscle imbalance Side dominance Forward shoulder posture Forward head posture
	Winging scapula	Poor posture Muscle imbalance Muscular weakness
Shoulder heights	Shoulder heights unequal	Scoliosis Dominant side Scapula positioning
Neck musculature	The upper trapezius hypertrophied in relation to other periscapula muscles	Overused in normal upper extremity activities or overemphasized in weight lifting Side dominance
Head position	The head not sitting in a vertical position in relation to the neck Side bend, rotated	Caused by muscle imbalance Poor postural, proprioceptive sense Compensation for scoliosis Torticollis (acquired or congenital)

STJ = subtalar joint.

Measuring Leg Length

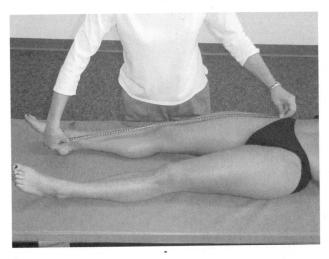

A

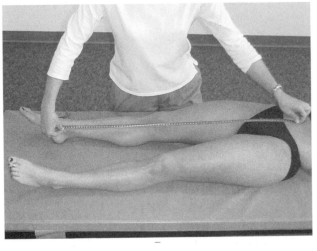

B

FIGURE 3–1 (A) Test for the presence of a structural (true) leg length discrepancy. Measurements are taken from the anterior superior iliac spine to the medial malleolus. Bilateral discrepancies of greater than $^1/_4$ inch are considered significant. (B) Test for the presence of a functional (apparent) leg length discrepancy. Measurements are taken from each medial malleolus to the umbilicus. This test is meaningful only if the test for a true leg length difference is negative.

Posture

Posture

Table 3–4 Leg Length Differences

Category Type	Description	Possible Causes
Functional or apparent leg length	Secondary to pelvic obliquity The asymmetry of the pelvis' altering the functional standing position and giving the appearance that one leg is longer or shorter than the other	Muscle weaknesses or imbalances around the pelvic region, unilateral hyperpronation of the foot, or any altered mechanics of the lower extremity
Structural or true leg length	Secondary to an actual difference in the length of the femur or the tibia of one leg compared with the other	Possibly from disruption in the growth plate of one of the long bones or a congenital anomaly
Compensatory leg length	A change in the joint angle of the foot, ankle, knee, or hip to compensate for other factors giving the appearance that one leg is longer than the other, yet they are equal	Factors such as pain, scoliosis, biomechanical changes

Box 3-3 Measured Block Method of Determining Leg Length Differences

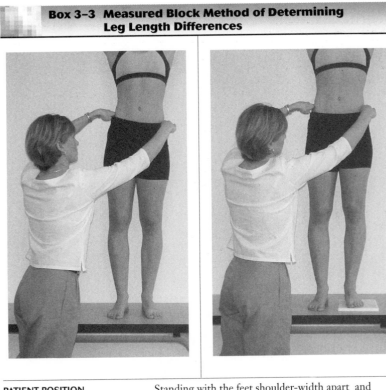

PATIENT POSITION	Standing with the feet shoulder-width apart and the weight evenly distributed
POSITION OF EXAMINER	Standing in front of the patient
EVALUATIVE PROCEDURE	The starting levels of the iliac crests are noted. Blocks of known thickness (measured in millimeters) are placed under the shorter leg until the iliac crests are of equal height. The leg length difference is calculated by totaling the sum of the heights of the individual blocks.
POSITIVE TEST	A leg length difference of greater than 0.7 cm (¼ in) is considered significant.
COMMENT	When the iliac crests are level, observe the heights of the ASIS. If the ASIS are not an equal height, then the patient has an asymmetrical pelvis.

ASIS = anterior superior iliac spine.

Posture

Box 3–4 Inspection of Pelvic Position

Neutral

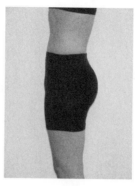

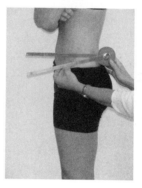

8 to 10° angle between the
ASIS and PSIS

ASIS = anterior superior iliac spine; PSIS = posterior superior iliac spine.

Box 3–4 Inspection of Pelvic Position (Continued)

Anterior Pelvic Tilt	Posterior Pelvic Tilt

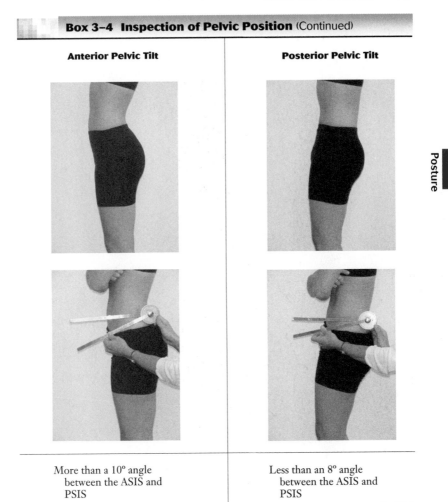

More than a 10° angle between the ASIS and PSIS	Less than an 8° angle between the ASIS and PSIS

ASIS = anterior superior iliac spine; PSIS = posterior superior iliac spine.

Posture

Posture

Box 3–5 Inspection of Scapular Posture

Scapular Elevation/Depression

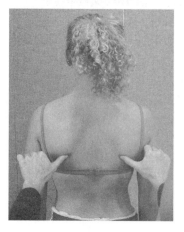

The height of the scapula are compared using the inferior angle as a landmark.

Scapular Protraction/Retraction

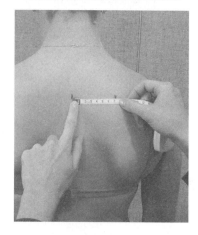

The distance from the T3 spinous process to the medial border of the scapula is measured. The normal value is 5 to 7 cm. An increased distance represents a protracted scapular position; a decreased distance, a retracted scapula.

Scapular Rotation

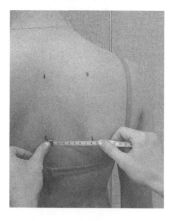

The distance from the T7 vertebrae to the inferior angle of each scapula is measured. An increased distance indicates an upwardly rotated scapula.

Scapular Winging

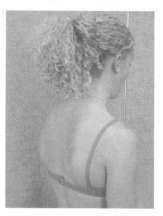

Elevation of the inferior angle of the scapula. Scapular tipping is characterized by the vertebral border lifting away from the thorax.

Box 3-6 Genu Recurvatum

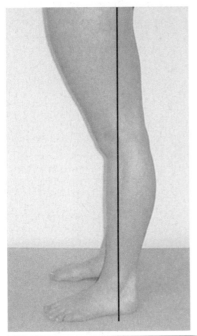

Possible causes	Hypermotility of joints/lax ligaments (commonly seen in ectomorph body type) Poor postural sense
Possible adverse effects	Increased stress on the ACL Increased tension on the posterior and posterolateral soft tissue structures Compressive forces on the anterior and medial compartments of the tibiofemoral joint

Posture

ACL = anterior cruciate ligament.

Box 3-7   Hyperlordotic Posture

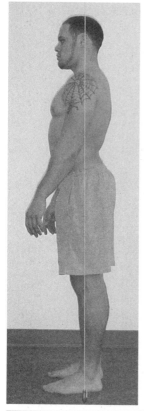

Joints involved	Lumbar spine, pelvis, hip
Possible cause	Tightened or shortened hip flexor muscles or back extensors Weakened or elongated hip extensors or abdominals Poor postural sense
Possible adverse effects	Increased lumbar lordosis Anterior pelvic tilt Hip assuming a flexed position
Possible associated compressive or distractive forces and pathological conditions	Increased shear forces placed on lumbar vertebral bodies secondary to psoas tightness Increased compressive forces on lumbar facet joints Adaptive shortening of the posterior lumbar spine ligaments and the anterior hip ligaments Elongation of the anterior lumbar spine ligaments and the posterior hip ligaments Narrowing of the lumbar intervertebral foramen

Box 3-8 Kypholordotic Posture

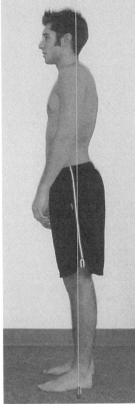

Joints involved	Pelvis, hip joint, lumbar spine, thoracic spine, cervical spine

Possible cause	Poor postural sense
	Muscle imbalance:
	  Tightened or shortened hip flexors or back extensors
	  Weakened or elongated hip extensors or trunk flexors

Possible adverse effects	Anterior pelvic tilt Hip joint flexion Increased lumbar lordosis (extension) Increased thoracic kyphosis (flexion)
Possible associated compressive or distractive forces and pathological conditions	Adaptive shortening of anterior chest musculature Elongation of thoracic paraspinal musculature Increased compressive forces on anterior structures of thoracic vertebrae and posterior structures of lumbar vertebrae Increased tensile forces on ligamentous structures in posterior aspect of thoracic spine and anterior aspect of lumbar spine Increased compression of lumbar facet joints Increased compression of thoracic anterior vertebral bodies Forward head posture Forward shoulder posture

Posture

Box 3-9 Swayback Posture

Joints involved	Knee joint, hip joint, lumbar spine, lower thoracic spine, cervical spine
Possible cause	Ectomorph body type: hypermobility of joints Poor postural sense Tightened or shortened hip extensors Weakened or elongated hip flexors or lower abdominals Decreased general muscular strength
Possible adverse effects	Genu recurvatum Hip joint extension Posterior pelvic tilt Anterior shift of the lumbosacral region Lumbar spine in neutral or minimal flexed position Increase in lower thoracic, thoracolumbar curvature (increase in lower thoracic kyphosis to cause posterior shift of trunk to compensate for anterior shift of L5/S1)
Possible associated compressive or distractive forces and pathological conditions	Elongation or increased tensile forces on the ligamentous structures at the anterior hip joint and posterior aspect of the lower thoracic spine Adaptively shortened or increased compressive forces on the posterior ligamentous structures at the hip joint and anterior aspect of the lower thoracic spine Increased tensile forces on the soft tissue structures of the posterior knee; compressive forces on anterior knee Result in increased stresses on joints; increased shearing forces L5/S1 Forward head posture Forward shoulder posture

Box 3-10   Flat Back Posture

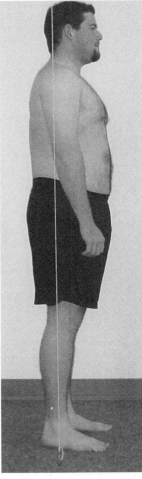

Joints involved	Hip joint, lumbar spine, thoracic spine, cervical spine
Possible causes	Shortened or tightened hip extensors, abdominal musculature Weakened/elongated hip flexors, back extensors Poor postural sense
Possible adverse effects	Extended hip joint Posterior pelvic tilt Flexed lumbar spine (decreased lumbar lordosis) Extended thoracic spine (decreased thoracic kyphosis) Flexed middle and lower cervical spine, extended upper cervical spine (FSP)
Possible associated compressive or distractive forces and pathological conditions	Adaptive shortening of soft tissue, compressive forces in posterior hip joint, anterior lumbar and mid-low cervical spines, posterior thoracic and upper cervical spines Elongation of soft tissue, tensile forces on the anterior hip joint, posterior lumbar and middle and lower cervical spines, anterior thoracic and upper cervical spines FHP resulting as compensation for the posterior displacement of the spine Knee flexion possibly occurring for the same reason

FHP = forward head posture; FSP = forward shoulder posture.

Posture

Box 3–11 Scoliosis

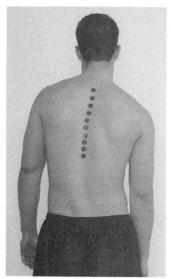

Joints involved	Thoracic and lumbar vertebrae
Possible causes	Structural scoliosis: Anomaly of vertebrae Functional scoliosis: Muscle imbalance, leg length discrepancy
Possible adverse effects	Rotation of one or more vertebrae Compresson of one facet joint; distraction of the opposite facet joint Shortened or tightened trunk muscles on concave side of the curvature Weakened or elongated trunk muscles on convex side of the curvature
Possible associated compressive or distractive forces and pathological conditions	Disk pathology Soft tissue pathology as the body attempts to compensate and maintain head posture Sacroiliac joint dysfunction Decreased mobility of spine and chest cage Asymmetry in chest expansion with deep breathing Decreased pulmonary function (if excessive in thoracic region) If caused by limb length inequality: Degenerative changes in lumbar spine, hip, knee joints in longer limb Muscle overuse on longer limb caused by increased muscle activity S-I joint dysfunction Excessive pronation of longer limb with dysfunctions associated with pronation Alteration of pattern of mechanical stresses on joint involved—structural

Box 3–12 Forward Shoulder Posture

Joints involved	Scapulothoracic articulation Glenohumeral joint Thoracic spine Cervical spine
Possible causes	Tightened, shortened, or overdeveloped anterior shoulder girdle muscles (pectoralis major, pectoralis minor) Weakened or elongated interscapula muscles (middle trap, rhomboid, lower trap) Poor postural awareness Abnormal cervical and thoracic spine sagittal plane arrangements Postural muscle fatigue Large breast development Repetitive occupational and sporting positions
Possible adverse effects	Humeral head is displaced anteriorly Forward head posture
Possible associated compressive or distractive forces and pathological conditions	Thoracic outlet syndrome Abnormal scapulohumeral rhythm and scapula stability Acromioclavicular degeneration Bicipital tendinitis Impingement syndrome Trigger points, myofascial pain in periscapular muscles Abnormal biomechanics of glenohumeral joint

Posture

Box 3–13   Forward Head Posture

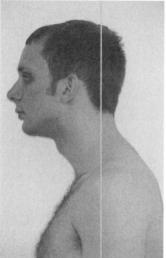

Joints involved	Cervical spine GH joint Thoracic spine
Possible causes	Wearing of bifocals Poor eyesight and need for glasses Muscle fatigue and weakness Poor postural sense Compensatory mechanism for other postural deviations (occupational activities and ADLs)
Possible adverse effects	Flexion of lower cervical spine Flattening or flexion of mid-cervical spine Extension of upper cervical spine Affects the normal GH joint motion
Possible associated compressive/distractive forces and pathological conditions	Adaptively shortened suboccipital muscles (capital extensors), scalenes, upper trapezius, and levator scapula Elongated and weakened anterior cervical flexors and scapular depressors Hypomobile upper cervical region with compensatory hypermobility of the mid-cervical spine Abnormal shoulder (GH joint) biomechanics; decrease in shoulder elevation Temporomandibular joint dysfunction Thoracic outlet syndrome involving the anterior and mid-scalene region Myofascial pain periscapula muscles and posterior cervical muscles[36] Muscle overuse of posterior cervical and upper shoulder girdle muscles to maintain head in forward posture Forward shoulder posture

ADLs = activities of daily living; GH = glenohumeral.

4

The Foot and Toes

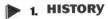
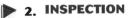
49

Map

50   CHAPTER 4   The Foot and Toes

Evaluation of the Foot and Toes (Continued)

Medial talar tubercle
Calcaneal dome
Flexor hallucis longus
Flexor digitorum longus
Tibialis posterior
Posterior tibial artery

Lateral Structures
Fifth MTP joint
Fifth metatarsal
Styloid process
Cuboid
Lateral border of the calcaneus
Peroneal tendons

Dorsal Structures
Sinus tarsi
Dome of the talus
Cuneiforms
Rays
Tibialis anterior
Extensor hallucis longus
Extensor digitorum longus
Extensor digitorum brevis
Inferior extensor retinaculum
Dorsalis pedal artery
Intermetatarsal neuromas

Plantar Structures
Medial calcaneal tubercle
Plantar fascia
Sesamoid bones of the great toe

Metatarsal Heads

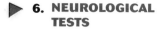 ## 4. RANGE OF MOTION TESTS

Toes Active ROM
Flexion
Extension

Toes Passive ROM
Flexion
Extension

Toes Resisted ROM
Flexion
Extension

Related Motions
Subtalar joint
Inversion
Eversion
Talocrural joint
Dorsiflexion
Plantarflexion

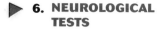 ## 5. LIGAMENTOUS CAPSULAR TESTS

MTP and IP Joints
Valgus stress testing
Varus stress testing

Metatarsal and Tarsal Joints
Intermetatarsal glide
Tarsometatarsal joint glide
Midtarsal joint glide
Mobility of the first ray

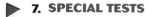 ## 6. NEUROLOGICAL TESTS

Tarsal Tunnel
Peroneal nerve
Sciatic nerve
Lumbar or sacral nerve root
impingement

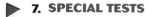 ## 7. SPECIAL TESTS

Arch Pathologies
Test for supple pes planus
Feiss' line
Navicular drop test

Tarsal Tunnel Syndrome
Tinel's sign

Metatarsal/Phalanx Fracture
Long bone compression test

Intermetatarsal Neuroma
Pencil test

IP = interphalangeal; MTP = metatarsophalangeal; ROM = range of motion.

Table 4–1 Possible Pathology Based on the Location of Pain

				Location of Pain		
	Proximal (Calcaneus)	Distal (Toes)	Plantar	Dorsal	Medial	Lateral
Soft tissue injury	Calcaneal bursitis Retrocalcaneal bursitis Achilles tendon inflammation	Corns Hallux rigidus IP sprain MTP sprain	Callus Plantar fasciitis Plantar fascia rupture Plantar warts Intermetatarsal neuroma Tarsal tunnel syndrome	MTP sprain Forefoot sprain	Medial arch pathology Plantar fasciitis Tarsal tunnel syndrome Tibialis posterior* Turf toe syndrome	Peroneal tendinitis*
Bony injury	Calcaneal fracture Calcaneal spur Calcaneal cyst	Phalanx fracture Arthritis or inflammation	Sesamoiditis Sesamoid fracture Heel spur	Metatarsal stress fracture Talus fracture Tarsal coalition	Navicular stress fracture Bunion Hallux rigidis	Cuboid fracture Fifth metatarsal fracture (especially at the base)

IP = interphalangeal; MTP = metatarsophalangeal.

Foot and Toes

52 CHAPTER 4 The Foot and Toes

Table 4-2 Summary of Non–Weight-Bearing and Weight-Bearing Subtalar Motions

Component Movements of Subtalar Supination/Pronation

Motion	Non–Weight Bearing	Weight Bearing
Supination	Calcaneal inversion (or varus)	Calcaneal inversion (or varus)
	Calcaneal adduction	Talar abduction (or lateral rotation)
	Calcaneal plantarflexion	Talar dorsiflexion
		Tibiofibular lateral rotation
Pronation	Calcaneal eversion (or valgus)	Calcaneal eversion (or valgus)
	Calcaneal abduction	Talar adduction (or medial rotation)
	Calcaneal dorsiflexion	Talar plantarflexion
		Tibiofibular medial rotation

Inspection

Inspection of Foot Posture

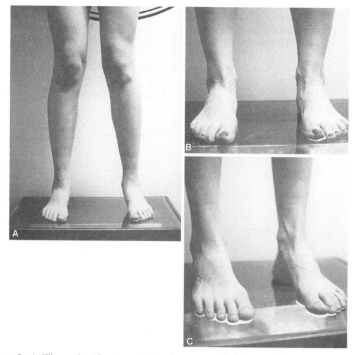

Figure 4–1 Three classifications of feet: **(A)** pronated, **(B)** normal, **(C)** supinated.

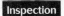

Table 4–3 Classification Scheme for the Clinical Definition of Foot Type (Weight Bearing)*

Pronated Foot	Supinated Foot
• The calcaneus must be everted greater than 3° from perpendicular relative to the position of the ground. • A medial bulge must be present at the talonavicular joint, indicating excessive talar adduction. • The medial arch must be low. This is determined by Feiss' line, formed by connecting the points formed by the head of the first metatarsal, the navicular tubercle, and the medial malleolus (see Box 4–2).	• The calcaneus must be inverted greater than 3° from perpendicular relative to the position of the ground. • A medial bulge must not be present at the talonavicular joint, indicating excessive talar adduction. • Using Feiss' line, the arch must be high.

*Each of the three criteria under each of the column headings must be met for the foot to be classified as such; otherwise, the foot should be categorized as neutral.

Adapted from Dahle, LK, et al: Visual assessment of foot type and relationship of foot type to lower extremity injury. J Orthop Sports Phys Ther 14:70, 1991.

Foot and Toes

Foot and Toes

Box 4–1 Pathological Toe Postures

Claw Toes	Hammer Toes

Observation

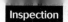

Illustration

Deviation

Contracture of the interosseous or lumbrical muscles (or both)

Contractures of the associated toe extensors and flexors; inability of the interosseous muscles to hold the proximal phalanx in the neutral position

Posture

Hyperextension of the MTP joint and flexion of the PIP and DIP joints. Claw toes affect the lateral four toes.

Hyperextension of the MTP and DIP joints and flexion of the PIP joints of the lateral four toes.

DIP = distal interphalangeal; PIP = proximal interphalangeal; MTP = metatarsophalangeal.

Box 4-1 Pathological Toe Postures (Continued)

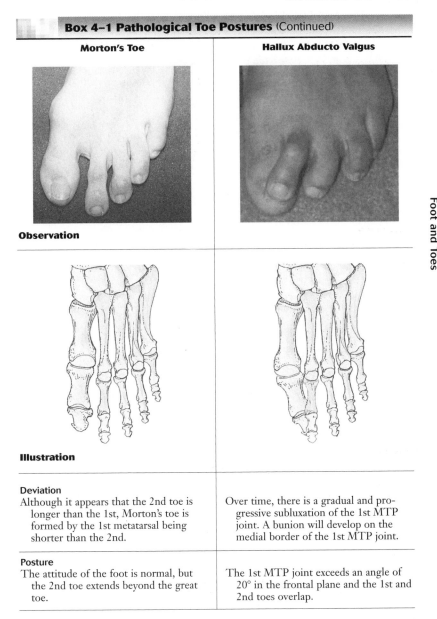

Morton's Toe	Hallux Abducto Valgus
Observation	
Illustration	

Deviation

Although it appears that the 2nd toe is longer than the 1st, Morton's toe is formed by the 1st metatarsal being shorter than the 2nd.

Over time, there is a gradual and progressive subluxation of the 1st MTP joint. A bunion will develop on the medial border of the 1st MTP joint.

Posture

The attitude of the foot is normal, but the 2nd toe extends beyond the great toe.

The 1st MTP joint exceeds an angle of 20° in the frontal plane and the 1st and 2nd toes overlap.

MTP = metatarsophalangeal.

Foot and Toes

PALPATION

Palpation of the Medial Structures

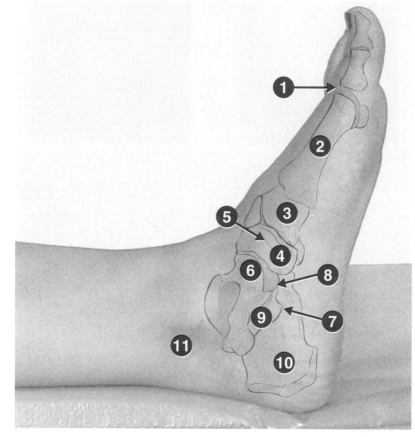

MEDIAL STRUCTURES

1 First MTP joint
2 First metatarsal
3 First cuneiform
4 Navicular
5 Navicular tuberosity
6 Talar head
7 Sustentaculum tali

8 Spring ligament
9 Medial talar tubercle
10 Calcaneus
11 Medial tendons: Flexor hallucis longus; flexor digitorum longus; tibialis posterior

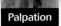
Palpation of the Lateral Structures

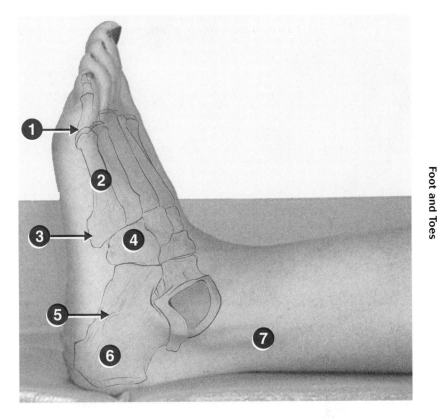

LATERAL STRUCTURES

1 Fifth MTP joint
2 Fifth metatarsal
3 Styloid tuberosity of 5th metatarsal
4 Cuboid

5 Peroneal tubercle
6 Lateral border of the calcaneus
7 Peroneal tendons

Palpation of the Dorsal Structures

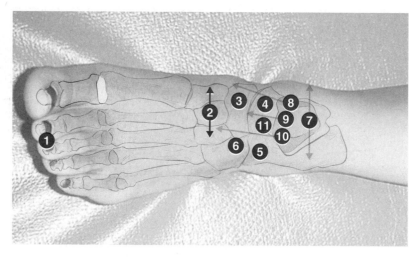

Dorsal Structures

1 Rays

2 Cuneifoms

3 Navicular

4 Dome of the talus

5 Sinus tarsi

6 Extensor digitorum brevis

7 Inferior extensor retinaculum

8 Tibialis anterior

9 Extensor hallucis longus

10 Extensor digitorum longus

11 Dorsalis pedis pulse

Foot and Toes

Palpation of the Plantar Structures

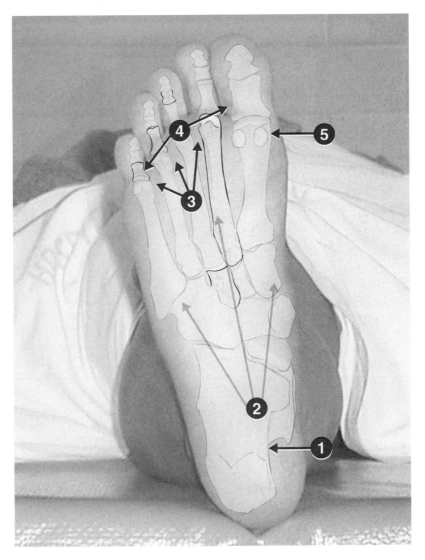

Foot and Toes

PLANTAR STRUCTURES
1 Medial calcaneal tubercle
2 Plantar fascia
3 Intermetatarsal neuromas
4 Metatarsal heads
5 Sesamoid bones of the first MTP joint

RANGE OF MOTION TESTING

Foot and Toes

Box 4–2 Foot Goniometry

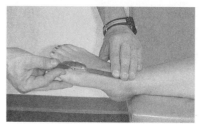 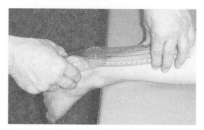

	Flexion and Extension (MTP, IP, PIP, and DIP)	Rearfoot (Subtalar) Inversion and Eversion
Patient Position	Supine	Prone
Goniometer Alignment		
Fulcrum	Positioned over the dorsal aspect of the joint being tested	Centered over the Achilles tendon with the axis bisecting the malleoli
Stationary Arm	Centered on the midline of the bone proximal to the joint being tested	Centered on the midline of the lower leg
Movement Arm	Centered on the midline of the bone distal to the joint being tested	Centered over the midline of the calcaneus

DIP = distal interphalangeal; IP = interphalangeal; PIP = proximal interphalangeal; MTP = metatarsophalangeal.

Table 4–4 Foot and Toes–Capsular Patterns and End-Feels

Midtarsal Joints
   Capsular Pattern: dorsiflexion, plantarflexion, adduction, internal rotation
Abduction Firm – Capsule and other soft tissue stretch
Adduction Firm – Capsule and other soft tissue stretch

Metatarsophalangeal Joints
   Capsular Pattern – 1st toe: extension, flexion
   Capsular Pattern – 2nd – 5th toes: flexion, extension

Interphalangeal Joints
   Capsular Pattern: flexion, extension
Flexion   Firm – Dorsal joint capsule; extensor digitorum brevis (first toe)
Extension Firm – Plantar joint capsule; flexor hallucis brevis; flexor digitorum brevis;
   flexor digiti minimi
Abduction Firm – Collateral ligament; web space
Adduction Firm/Hard – Collateral ligament; approximation with medial toe

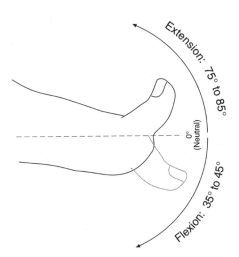

Figure 4–2 Active range of motion for flexion and extension of the great toe's metatarsophalangeal (MTP) joint. The range of motion decreases with each subsequent joint from the first MTP joint to the fifth.

Foot and Toes

62   C H A P T E R 4   The Foot and Toes

Box 4–3 Resisted Range of Motion for the Toes

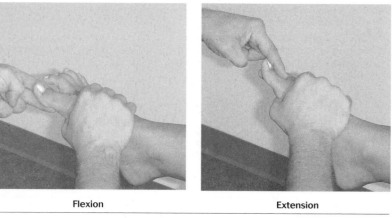

Flexion	Extension

STARTING POSITION	The joint being tested is placed in the neutral position	
STABILIZATION	The forefoot is stabilized by grasping the metatarsals proximal to their heads.	
RESISTANCE	**Great toe:** along the entire length of the toe's plantar aspect **Lateral four toes:** on their plantar aspect	**Great toe:** along the entire length of the toe's dorsal aspect **Lateral four toes:** on their dorsal aspect
MUSCLES TESTED	**Great toe:** Flexor hallucis longus, flexor hallucis brevis **Lateral four toes:** Flexor digitorum longus, flexor digitorum brevis, flexor digiti minimi brevis, dorsal interossei (MTP joint flexion), plantar interossei (MTP joint flexion), lumbricals (MTP flexion)	**Great toe:** Extensor hallucis longus, extensor hallucis brevis **Lateral four toes:** Extensor digitorum longus, extensor digitorum brevis, dorsal interossei (IP joint extension), plantar interossei (IP joint extension), lumbricals (IP joint extension)

IP = interphalangeal; MTP = metatarsophalangeal.

Ligamentous and Capsular Testing

Box 4–4 Valgus and Varus Stress Testing of the MTP and IP Joints

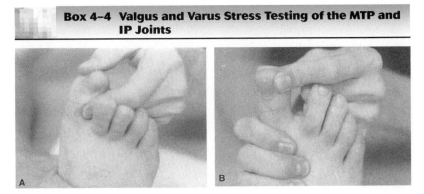

Stress testing of the toe's capsular ligaments: **(A)** Valgus stress applied to the interphalangeal joint; **(B)** varus stress applied to the MTP joint.

PATIENT POSITION	Supine or sitting
POSITION of EXAMINER	Standing The proximal bone stabilized close to the joint to be tested The bone distal to the joint being tested grasped near the middle of its shaft Care is necessary to isolate the joint being tested.
EVALUATIVE PROCEDURE	**Valgus testing (A):** The distal bone is moved laterally, attempting to open up the joint on the medial side. **Varus testing (B):** The distal bone is moved medially, attempting to open up the joint on the lateral side.
POSITIVE TEST	Pain or increased laxity when compared with the same joint on the opposite extremity
IMPLICATIONS	**Valgus test (A):** MCL sprain of the involved joint **Varus test (B):** LCL sprain of the involved joint

IP = interphalangeal; LCL = lateral collateral ligament; MCL = medial collateral ligament; MTP = metatarsophalangeal.

Foot and Toes

Box 4–5 Intermetatarsal Glide Test

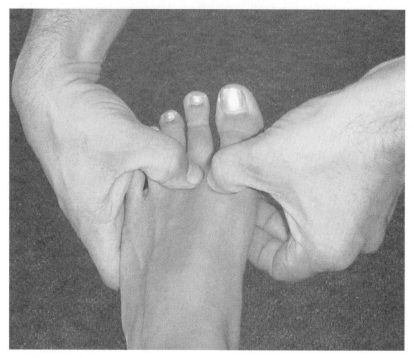

Assessment of the amount of intermetatarsal glide between the 1st and 2nd metatarsal heads. Perform this test for each of the four articulations formed between the five metatarsals.

PATIENT POSITION	Supine or sitting on the table with the knees extended
POSITION OF EXAMINER	Standing in front of the patient's feet One hand grasping the first MT head; the other grasping the second MT head
EVALUATIVE PROCEDURE	The two MT heads are moved in opposite directions (plantarly and dorsally and then dorsally and plantarly). This procedure is repeated by moving to the lateral MT heads until all four intermetatarsal joints have been evaluated.
POSITIVE TEST	Pain or increased glide compared with the opposite extremity
IMPLICATIONS	Trauma to the deep transverse metatarsal ligament, interosseous ligament, or both Pain without the presence of laxity may indicate the presence of a neuroma

MT = metatarsal.

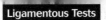

Box 4–6 Tarsometatarsal Joint Glides

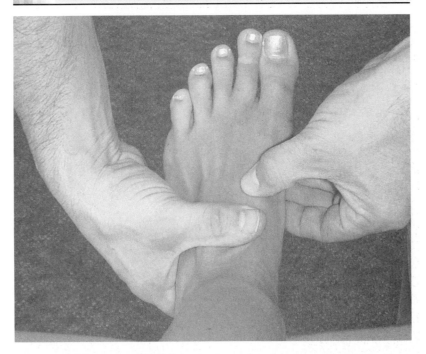

Assessment of the amount of glide between the tarsals and the base of the metatarsals. Perform this test on each of the five tarsometatarsal joints.

PATIENT POSITION	Supine Knee flexed and the heel stabilized by the edge of the table
POSITION OF EXAMINER	Standing or sitting in front of the patient's foot One hand grasping the distal tarsal row The opposite hand grasping the metatarsal being glided
EVALUATIVE PROCEDURE	The metatarsal is glided dorsally on the tarsal and then glided plantarly on the tarsal. Repeat for each joint
POSITIVE TEST	Pain associated with movement Increased or decreased glide relative to the opposite foot
IMPLICATIONS	Increased glide: ligamentous laxity Decreased glide: joint adhesions, articular changes causing coalition of the joint

Box 4–7 Midtarsal Joint Glides

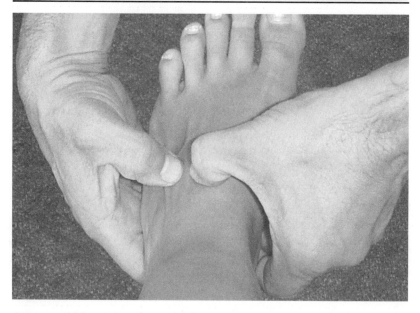

Assessment of the amount of joint glide between the tarsals.

PATIENT POSITION	Supine Knee flexed and the heel stabilized by the edge of the table
POSITION OF EXAMINER	Standing or sitting in front of the patient's foot Grasp the plantar and dorsal aspect of one tarsal with the stabilizing hand. The opposite hand grasps the adjacent tarsal in a similar manner
EVALUATIVE PROCEDURE	One tarsal is glided dorsally and then plantarly on the stabilized tarsal Repeat for each tarsal joint
POSITIVE TEST	Pain associated with movement Increased or decreased glide relative to the opposite foot
IMPLICATIONS	Increased glide: ligamentous laxity Decreased glide: joint adhesions, articular changes causing coalition of the joint

SPECIAL TESTS

Box 4–8 Feiss' Line for Navicular Drop

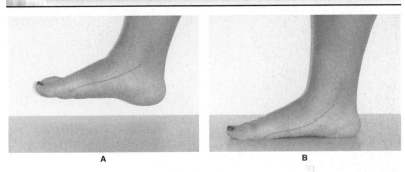

A   **B**

With the patient in a non–weight-bearing position, a line is drawn from the apex of the medial malleolus and the plantar aspect of the 1st MTP joint. The displacement of the navicular tubercle is marked when the patient bears weight.

PATIENT POSITION	Sitting with the feet off the end of the table
POSITION OF EXAMINER	Positioned at the patient's feet
EVALUATIVE PROCEDURE	With the patient non–weight bearing, the examiner identifies and marks the apex of the medial malleolus and the plantar aspect of the 1st MTP joint. A line is drawn connecting the marks over the first MTP joint and the medial malleolus (**A**). Mark the position of the navicular tubercle. The patient stands with the feet approximately 1 ft apart and the weight evenly distributed. The examiner should check that the line drawn previously still connects the apex of the medial malleolus and the plantar aspect of the first MTP joint. The new position of the navicular tubercle is marked (**B**).
POSITIVE TEST RESULT	A navicular that drops two thirds or greater the distance to the floor
IMPLICATIONS	Hyperpronated foot

MTP = metatarsophalangeal.

Foot and Toes

Box 4–9   Test for Supple Pes Planus

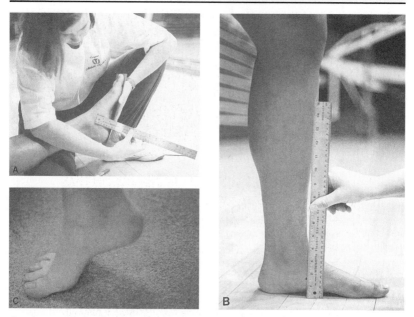

Supple pes planus. The patient displays a normal arch in the non–weight-bearing position **(A)**. In weight bearing, the arch disappears (ruler added for demonstrative purposes) **(B)**. When the patient performs a toe raise, the arch returns by means of the windlass effect **(C)**.

PATIENT POSITION	Sitting on the edge of the examination table
POSITION OF EXAMINER	Positioned at the patient's foot
EVALUATIVE PROCEDURE	With the patient in a non–weight-bearing position the examiner notes the presence of a medial longitudinal arch **(A)**. The examiner instructs the patient to stand so that the body weight is evenly distributed **(B)**.
POSITIVE TEST	The presence of a medial longitudinal arch when non–weight bearing disappears when weight bearing To confirm the presence of supple pes planus, note if the arch reappears as the patient performs a toe raise **(C)**.
IMPLICATIONS	If the medial longitudinal arch disappears when weight bearing, a supple pes planus is present. If no arch is present while in a non–weight-bearing position, a rigid pes planus is present.
COMMENT	This test is only meaningful when the medial longitudinal arch is present with the patient in a non–weight-bearing position.

Box 4–10 Navicular Drop Test

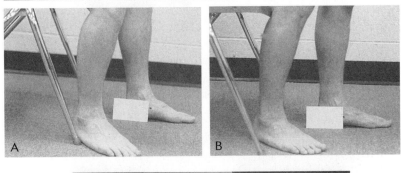

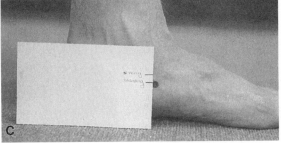

The navicular drop test is used to assess hyperpronation of the foot by measuring the height of the navicular tuberosity while the foot is non–weight-bearing (**A**) to weight bearing (**B**) and measuring the distance of the inferior displacement (**C**).

PATIENT POSITION	Sitting with both feet on the floor. A noncarpeted surface is recommended.
POSITION OF EXAMINER	Kneeling in front of the patient.
EVALUATIVE PROCEDURE	The subtalar joint is placed in the neutral position with the patient's foot flat against the ground, but non–weight-bearing. With the patient non–weight-bearing, a dot is placed over the navicular tuberosity. A 3 × 5 index card is positioned next to the medial longitudinal arch. A mark is made on the card corresponding to the level of the navicular tuberosity (**A**). The patient stands with the body weight evenly distributed between the two feet, and the foot is allowed to relax into pronation. The new level of the navicular is marked on the index card (**B**). The relative displacement (drop) of the navicular is determined by measuring the distance between the two marks in millimeters (**C**).
POSITIVE TEST	The navicular drops greater than 10 mm.
IMPLICATIONS	Hyperpronated foot.

Tinel's Sign for Tarsal Tunnel Syndrome

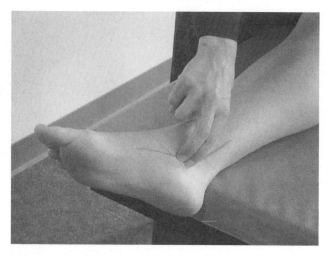

Figure 4–3 Location of Tinel's sign for tarsal tunnel syndrome. Tapping over the path of the posterior tibial nerve refers pain into the foot and toes.

Long Bone Compression Test

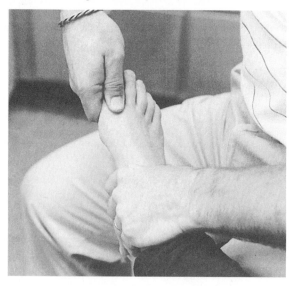

Figure 4–4 Long bone compression test for suspected fractures of the metatarsals. A longitudinal force is placed along the shaft of the bone. In the presence of a fracture, compression of the two fragments results in pain and possibly the presence of a "false joint."

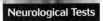

Test for Intermetatarsal Neuroma

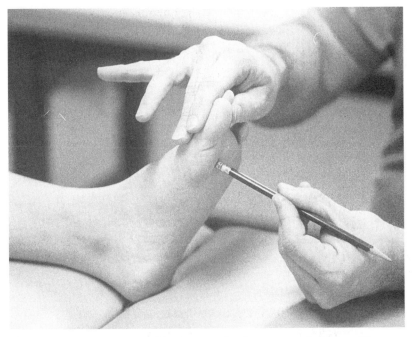

Figure 4–5 Determination of the presence of an intermetatarsal neuroma. The eraser end of a pencil is used to apply pressure to the intermetatarsal space, compressing the nerve ending.

Neurological Examination

Neurological Symptoms in the Foot

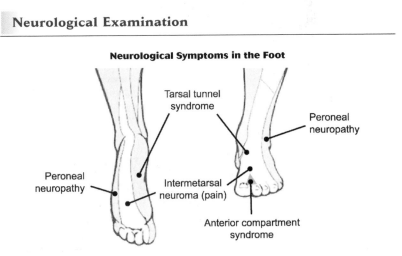

Figure 4–6 Peripheral neurological symptoms in the foot.

5

The Ankle and Lower Leg

EVALUATION MAP:
The Ankle and Lower Leg

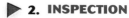

▶ 1. HISTORY

Location of the Pain
Nature or type of pain
Onset
Injury mechanisms
Level of activity and conditioning
   regimen
History of injury

▶ 2. INSPECTION

General Inspection
Weight-bearing status
General bilateral comparison
Swelling

Lateral Structures
Peroneal muscle group
Distal one-third of the fibula
Lateral malleolus

Anterior Structures
Appearance of the lower leg
Contour of the malleoli
Talus
Sinus tarsi

Medial Structures
Medial malleolus
Medial longitudinal arch

Posterior Structures
Gastrocnemius–soleus complex
Achilles tendon

Bursae
Calcaneus

▶ 3. PALPATION

Lateral Structures
Fibular shaft
Interosseous membrane
Anterior and posterior tibiofibular
   ligament
Calcaneofibular ligament
Anterior talofibular ligament
Posterior talofibular ligament
Peroneal tubercle
Cuboid
Base of the 5th metatarsal
Peroneus longus and brevis
Peroneal retinaculum

Anterior Structures
Anterior tibial shaft
Dome of the talus
Extensor retinacula
Sinus tarsi
Tibialis anterior
Long toe extensors
Peroneus tertius

Medial Structures
Medial malleolus
Deltoid ligament
Sustentaculum tali
Spring ligament
Navicular and navicular tubercle

CHAPTER 5

The Ankle and Lower Leg (Continued)

Talar head
Tibialis posterior
Long toe flexors

Posterior Structures
Gastrocnemius–soleus complex
Achilles tendon
Subtendinous calcaneal bursa
Subcutaneous calcaneal bursa
Dome of the calcaneus

Palpation of Pulses
Posterior tibial artery
Dorsalis pedis artery

▶ **4. RANGE OF MOTION TESTS**

AROM
Plantarflexion and dorsiflexion
Inversion and eversion

PROM
Plantarflexion and dorsiflexion
Inversion and eversion

RROM
Dorsiflexion
Plantarflexion
   Gastrocnemius
   Soleus
Inversion
Eversion

▶ **5. LIGAMENTOUS TESTS**

Anterior Talofibular Ligament Instability
Anterior drawer test

Calcaneofibular Ligament Instability
Inversion stress test (talar tilt)

Ankle Syndesmosis Instability
Kleiger's test
Squeeze test

Deltoid Ligament Instability
Eversion stress test (talar tilt)
External rotation test

▶ **6. NEUROLOGICAL TESTS**

Anterior compartment syndrome
Peroneal nerve involvement
Sciatic nerve involvement
Lumbar nerve root involvement

▶ **7. SPECIAL TESTS**

Lower Leg Fractures
Squeeze test

Stress Fracture
Bump test

Achilles Tendon Pathology
Thompson's test

Ankle and Lower Leg

AROM = active range of motion; PROM = passive range of motion; RROM = resisted range of motion.

History

Table 5–1 Possible Trauma Based on the Location of Pain (Excluding Gross Injury)

| | Location of Pain | | | |
	Lateral	Anterior	Medial	Posterior
Soft tissue	Inversion ankle sprain	Extensor retinaculum sprain	Evasion ankle sprain	Triceps surae strain
	Syndesmosis sprain	Syndesmosis sprain	Capsular impingement	Achilles tendinitis
	Capsular impingement	Tibialis anterior or long toe extensor strain	Tibialis posterior strain	Achilles tendon rupture
	Subluxating peroneal tendons	Tibialis anterior or long toe extensor tendinitis	Tibialis posterior tendinitis	Subtendinous calcaneal bursitis
	Peroneal muscle strain	Anterior compartment syndrome		Subcutaneous calcaneal bursitis
	Peroneal tendinitis	Interosseous membrane trauma		Deep vein thrombophlebitis
	Interosseous membrane trauma	Anterior tibiofibular ligament sprain		Posterior tibiofibular ligament sprain
	Peroneal nerve trauma			
Bony	Lateral ligament avulsion	Tibial stress fracture	Medial ligament avulsion	Calcaneal fracture
	Lateral malleolus fracture	Talar fracture	Medial malleolus avulsion	Arthritis
	Fibular stress fracture	Talar osteochondritis	Medial malleolus fracture	Os trigonum trauma
	Fifth MT fracture	Arthritis	Arthritis	
	Peroneal tendon avulsion	Periosteitis		
	Arthritis			

MT = metatarsal.

Table 5-2 Mechanism of Ankle Injury and the Resultant Tissue Damage

Uniplanar Motion	Tensile Forces	Compressive Forces
Inversion	Lateral structures: Anterior talofibular ligament, calcaneofibular ligament, posterior talofibular ligament, lateral capsule, and peroneal tendons; lateral malleolus fracture	Medial structures: Medial malleolus, deltoid ligament, and medial neurovascular bundle
Eversion	Medial structures: Deltoid ligament, tibialis posterior, and long toe flexors	Lateral structures: Lateral malleolus and lateral capsule
Plantarflexion	Anterior structures: Anterior capsule, long toe extensors, and extensor retrinaculum Lateral structures: Anterior talofibular ligament	Posterior structures: Posterior capsule, subtendinous calcaneal bursa, subcutaneous calcaneal bursa, os trigonum, and talus fracture
Dorsiflexion	Posterior structures: Triceps surae, Achilles tendon Lateral structures: Posterior talofibular ligament	Anterior structures: Anterior capsule, syndesmosis, and extensor retinaculum

Ankle and Lower Leg

PALPATION

Palpation of the Fibular Structures

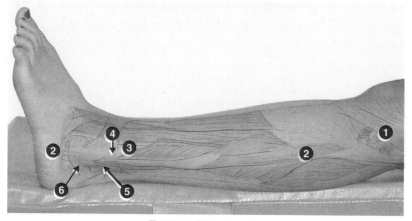

FIBULAR STRUCTURES

1 Common peroneal nerve
2 Peroneus longus and brevis
3 Fibular shaft

4 Anterior and posterior tibiofibular ligament
5 Interosseous membrane
6 Superior peroneal retinaculum

Palpation of the Lateral Ankle

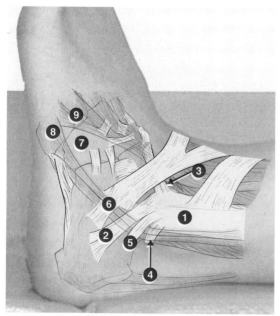

LATERAL ANKLE

1 Lateral malleolus
2 Calcaneofibular ligament
3 Anterior talofibular
4 Posterior talofibular ligament
5 Peroneal retinaculum
6 Peroneal tubercle
7 Cuboid
8 Base of the fifth metatarsal
9 Peroneus tertius

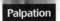

Palpation of the Anterior Structures

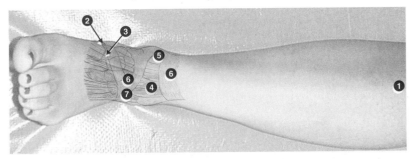

ANTERIOR ANKLE AND LEG

1 Anterior tibial shaft
2 Tibialis anterior
3 Extensor hallucis longus
4 Extensor digitorum longus
5 Dome of the talus
6 Extensor retinacula
7 Sinus tarsi

Palpation of the Medial Structures

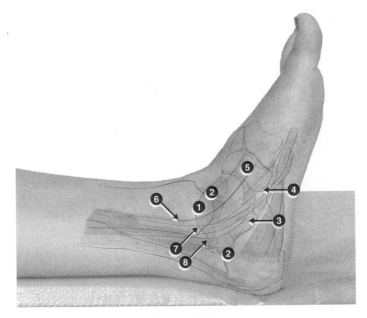

MEDIAL ANKLE

1 Medial malleolus
2 Deltoid ligament
3 Sustentaculum tali
4 Spring ligament
5 Navicular and navicular tuberosity
6 Tibialis posterior
7 Flexor digitorum longus
8 Flexor hallucis longus

Ankle and Lower Leg

Palpation of the Posterior Structures

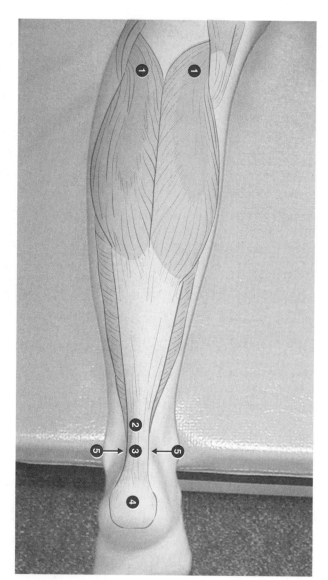

POSTERIOR STRUCTURE

1 Gastrocnemius-soleus complex
2 Achilles tendon
3 Subcutaneous calcaneal bursa
4 Calcaneus
5 Subtendinous calcaneal bursa

Range of Motion Testing

Box 5-1 Goniometry: Ankle

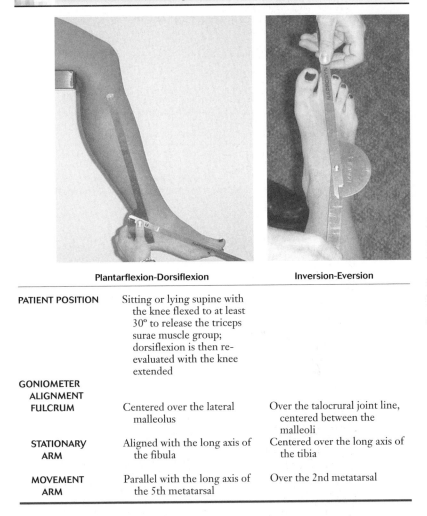

Plantarflexion-Dorsiflexion	Inversion-Eversion

	Plantarflexion-Dorsiflexion	**Inversion-Eversion**
PATIENT POSITION	Sitting or lying supine with the knee flexed to at least 30° to release the triceps surae muscle group; dorsiflexion is then re-evaluated with the knee extended	
GONIOMETER ALIGNMENT		
FULCRUM	Centered over the lateral malleolus	Over the talocrural joint line, centered between the malleoli
STATIONARY ARM	Aligned with the long axis of the fibula	Centered over the long axis of the tibia
MOVEMENT ARM	Parallel with the long axis of the 5th metatarsal	Over the 2nd metatarsal

Ankle and Lower Leg

Table 5–3 Ankle and Lower Leg–Capsular Patterns and End-Feels

Talocrural Joint
  Capsular Pattern: plantarflexion, dorsiflexion

Plantarflexion	Firm–Anterior joint capsule and ligaments; tibialis anterior; extensor hallucis longus; extensor digitorum longus
	Hard–Bony block between the talus and posterior tibia
Dorsiflexion	Firm–Achilles tendon; posterior capsule and ligaments

Subtalar Joint
  Capsular Pattern: inversion, eversion (varus, valgus)

Inversion	Firm–Calcaneofibular ligament; anterior talofibular ligament; posterior talofibular ligament; peroneal muscles
Eversion	Hard–Calcaneus and talus contacting the lateral malleolus
	Firm–Deltoid ligament; tibialis posterior

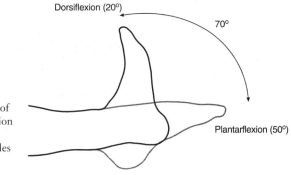

**Ankle Range of Motion:
Talocrural Plantarflexion and Dorsiflexion**

Dorsiflexion (20°)

70°

Plantarflexion (50°)

Figure 5–1 Range of motion for plantarflexion and dorsiflexion. Tightness of the Achilles tendon limits dorsiflexion.

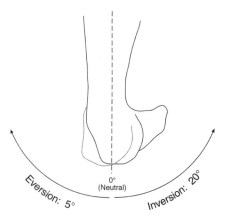

**Ankle Range of Motion:
Subtalar Inversion and Eversion**

0°
(Neutral)

Eversion: 5°

Inversion: 20°

Figure 5–2 Range of motion for inversion and eversion.

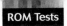
Isolating the Soleus

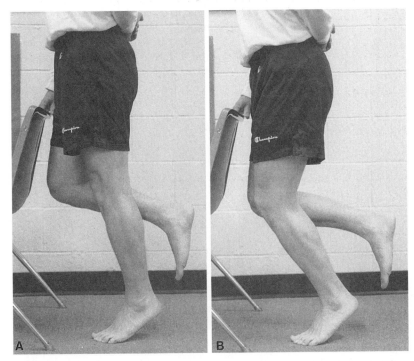

Figure 5–3 Toe-raise test for plantarflexion. (**A**) With the knee extended to include the gastrocnemius. (**B**) With the knee flexed to isolate the soleus muscle.

Ankle and Lower Leg

Box 5-2   Resisted Ankle Range of Motion

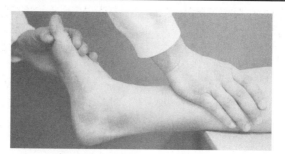

Dorsiflexion

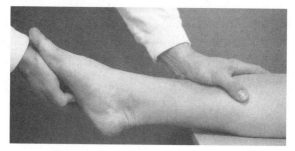

	Dorsiflexion	Plantarflexion
STARTING POSITION	Plantarflexion or neutral	Dorsiflexion or neutral; extend the knee to check the triceps surae as a group; flex the knee to at least 30° to isolate the soleus
STABILIZATION	Anterior aspect of the distal lower leg	Anterior aspect of the distal lower leg
RESISTANCE	Dorsum of the foot	Plantar aspect of the foot
SUBSTITUTION	Extension of the toes indicates that the extensor digitorum longus or extensor hallucis longus is contributing to the motion	Inversion of the foot indicates that the tibialis posterior, flexor digitorum longus, and/or flexor hallucis longus is contributing to the motion.
MUSCLES TESTED	Tibialis anterior, extensor digitorum longus, extensor hallucis longus, peroneus tertius	Gastrocnemius, soleus, tibialis posterior, peroneus longus, peroneus brevis, plantaris, flexor hallucis longus

Ankle and Lower Leg

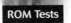

Box 5–2 Resisted Ankle Range of Motion (Continued)

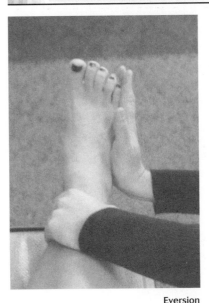 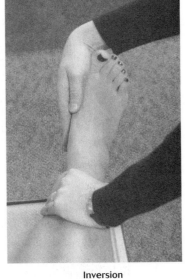

	Eversion	Inversion
STARTING POSITION	Inversion or neutral	Eversion or neutral
STABILIZATION	Distal lower leg	Distal lower leg
RESISTANCE	Lateral aspect of the foot	Medial aspect of the foot
SUBSTITUTION		Flexion of the toes could indicate substitution of the flexor hallucis longus or flexor digitorum longus muscles for the tibialis posterior
MUSCLES TESTED	Peroneus longus, peroneus brevis, extensor digitorum longus, peroneus tertius	Tibialis anterior, tibialis posterior, flexor hallucis longus, flexor digitorum longus

Ankle and Lower Leg

Tests for Ligamentous Stability

Box 5-3 Anterior Drawer Test

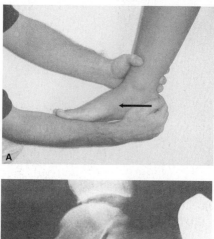

(A) Anterior drawer test to check the integrity of the anterior talofibular ligament.

(B) Radiographic view of a positive anterior drawer test. Note the anterior displacement of the talus relative to the tibia.

PATIENT POSITION	Sitting over the edge of the table with the knee flexed to prevent gastrocnemius tightness from influencing the outcome of the test.
POSITION OF EXAMINER	Sitting in front of the patient One hand stabilizes the lower leg, taking care not to occlude the mortise. The other hand cups the calcaneus while the forearm supports the foot in a position of slight plantarflexion.
EVALUATIVE PROCEDURE	The calcaneus and talus are drawn forward while providing a stabilizing force to the tibia.
POSITIVE TEST	The talus slides anteriorly from under the ankle mortise compared with the opposite side (assuming it is normal). There may be an appreciable "clunk" as the talus subluxates and relocates, or the patient may describe pain.
IMPLICATIONS	Tear of the anterior talofibular ligament and the associated capsule
MODIFICATION	The test may be performed with the patient supine, but the knee must be kept in a minimum of 30° flexion to eliminate the influence of the gastrocnemius muscle.

Ankle and Lower Leg

Box 5–4 Inversion Stress Test (Talar Tilt) (Continued)

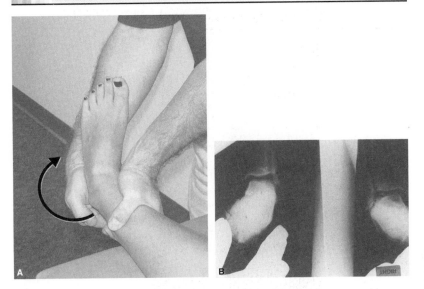

(A) Inversion stress test (talar tilt test) to check the integrity of the calcaneofibular ligament
(B) Radiograph of an inversion stress

PATIENT POSITION	Lying or sitting with legs over the edge of a table
POSITION OF EXAMINER	In front of the patient One hand grasps the calcaneus and maintains the foot and ankle in neutral position The opposite hand stabilizes the lower leg; the thumb or forefinger is placed along the calcaneofibular ligament so that any gapping of the talus away from the mortise can be felt.
EVALUATIVE PROCEDURE	The hand holding the calcaneus provides an inversion stress by rolling the calcaneus medially, causing the talus to tilt.
POSITIVE TEST	The talus tilts or gaps excessively, compared with the uninjured side; or pain is produced.
IMPLICATIONS	Involvement of the calcaneofibular ligament, possibly along with the anterior talofibular and posterior talofibular ligament

Box 5–5 Eversion Stress Test (Talar Tilt)

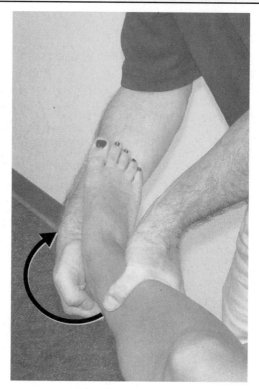

Eversion stress test to determine the integrity of the deltoid ligament, especially the tibiocalcaneal ligament

PATIENT POSITION	Lying or sitting with legs over the edge of a table
POSITION OF EXAMINER	In front of the patient One hand grasps the calcaneus and maintains the foot in a neutral position.
EVALUATIVE PROCEDURE	The opposite hand stabilizes the lower leg. The thumb or forefinger may be placed along the deltoid ligament so that any gapping of the talus away from the mortise can be felt. The hand holding the calcaneus rolls it laterally, tilting the talus and causing a gap on the medial side of the ankle mortise.
POSITIVE TEST	The talus tilts or gaps excessively as compared with the uninjured side, or pain is described during this motion.
IMPLICATIONS	The deltoid ligament has been compromised.

Box 5–6   External Rotation Test (Kleiger's Test)

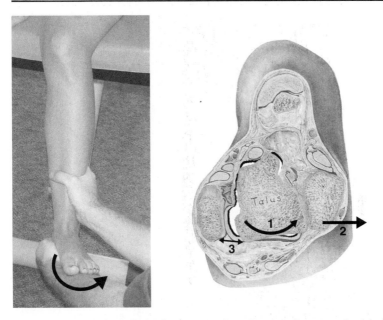

External rotation (Kleiger's) test for determination of rotatory damage to the deltoid ligament or the distal tibiofibular syndesmosis. The implication is based on the area of pain that is elicited.

Externally rotating the talus (**1**) places a lateral force on the fibula (**2**), spreading the syndesmosis and stretching the deltoid ligament (**3**).

PATIENT POSITION	Sitting with legs over the edge of the table
POSITION OF EXAMINER	In front of the patient One hand stabilizes the lower leg in a manner that does not compress the distal tibiofibular syndesmosis. The other hand grasps the medial aspect of the foot while supporting the ankle in a neutral position.
EVALUATIVE PROCEDURE	The foot is externally rotated. To stress the syndesmosis, place the ankle in dorsiflexion. To stress the deltoid ligament, place the ankle in neutral position or slightly plantarflexed.
POSITIVE TEST	Deltoid ligament involvement: medial joint pain. The examiner may feel displacement of the talus away from the medial malleolus. Syndesmosis involvement: pain is described in the anterolateral ankle at the site of the distal tibiofibular syndesmosis.
IMPLICATIONS	Medial pain is indicative of trauma to the deltoid ligament. Pain in the area of the anterolateral ankle should be considered syndesmosis pathology unless determined otherwise (e.g., malleolus fracture)

Ankle and Lower Leg

SPECIAL TESTS

Box 5-7 Squeeze Test

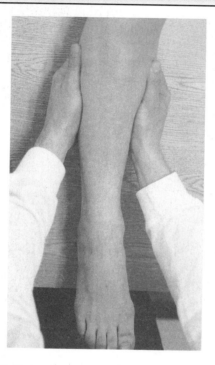

Squeeze test to identify fibular fractures or syndesmosis sprains. Pressure is applied transversely through the leg away from the site of pain.

PATIENT POSITION	Lying with the knee extended
POSITION OF EXAMINER	Standing next to, or in front of, the injured leg; the evaluator's hands cupped behind the tibia and fibula away from the site of pain
EVALUATIVE PROCEDURE	Gently squeeze (compress) the fibula and tibia, gradually adding more pressure if no pain or other symptoms are elicited. Progress toward the injured site until pain is elicited.
POSITIVE TEST	Pain is elicited, especially when it is away from the compressed area.
IMPLICATIONS	(A) Gross fracture or stress fracture of the fibula when pain is described along the fibular shaft (B) Syndesmosis sprain when pain is described at the distal tibiofibular joint
COMMENTS	Avoid applying too much pressure too soon into the test. Pressure should be applied gradually and progressively

Ankle and Lower Leg

Box 5–8 Bump Test for Lower Leg Stress Fractures

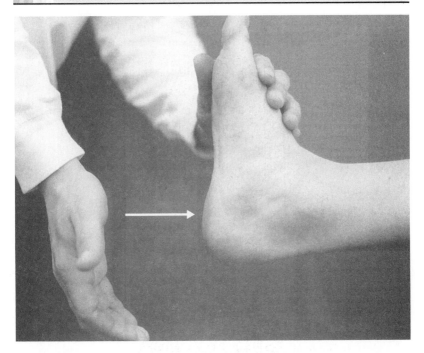

Bump test to identify stress fractures of the lower leg or talus. The examiner's hand is bumped against the patient's foot. The subsequent shock elicits pain in areas of stress fractures. Note that this test is not definitive.

PATIENT POSITION	Sitting with the involved leg off the end of the table and the knee straight, or lying supine The ankle in the neutral position
POSITION OF EXAMINER	Standing in front of the heel of the involved leg The posterior portion of the lower leg stabilized with the nondominant hand
EVALUATIVE PROCEDURE	Using the palm of the dominant hand, the examiner bumps the calcaneus with progressively more force until pain is elicited
POSITIVE TEST	Pain emanating from fracture of the calcaneus, talus, fibula, or tibia
IMPLICATIONS	Possible advanced stress fracture

Ankle and Lower Leg

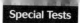
Ankle and Lower Leg

Box 5-9 Thompson's Test for Achilles Tendon Rupture

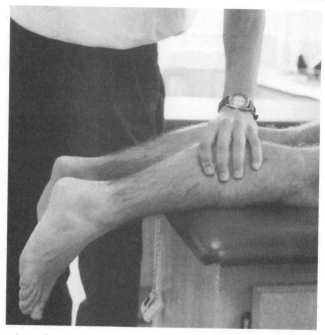

Thompson's test for an Achilles tendon rupture. When the Achilles tendon is intact, squeezing the calf muscle results in slight plantarflexion. A positive Thompson test occurs when the calf is squeezed but no motion is produced in the foot, indicating a tear of the Achilles tendon.

PATIENT POSITION	Prone, with the foot off the edge of the table
POSITION OF EXAMINER	At the side of the patient with one hand over the muscle belly of the calf musculature
EVALUATIVE PROCEDURE	The examiner squeezes the calf musculature while observing for plantarflexion of the foot
POSITIVE TEST	When the calf is squeezed, the foot does not plantarflex
IMPLICATIONS	The Achilles tendon has been ruptured

Box 5-10 Homan's Sign for Deep Vein Thrombosis

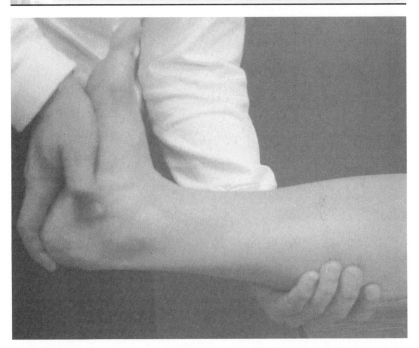

Homan's test for deep vein thrombosis. The calf is squeezed while the ankle is passively dorsiflexed. Indication of a positive result is a burning pain within the calf.

PATIENT POSITION	Sitting or supine with the knee extended
POSITION OF EXAMINER	At the end of the patient's leg with one hand on the plantar surface of the foot and the opposite hand grasping the calf.
EVALUATIVE PROCEDURE	The foot is passively dorsiflexed while the knee is kept extended. The examiner then squeezes the calf muscles.
POSITIVE TEST	Pain in the calf
IMPLICATIONS	Possible deep vein thrombophlebitis, this should be in agreement with other clinical findings of pain with deep palpation, swelling, heat, and dysfunction Ultrasonic imaging is used to make a definitive diagnosis of deep vein thrombosis.
NOTE	A strain of the gastrocnemius or soleus may produce a false-positive result with this examination.

Neurological Testing

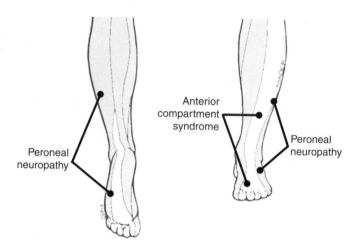

Figure 5-4 Local neuropathies of the ankle and lower leg. These findings should also be matched with those of a lower-quarter neurological screen.

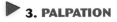

The Knee

EVALUATION MAP: The Knee

▶ 1. HISTORY

Location of pain
Mechanism of injury
Foot fixation
Associated sounds or sensations
Onset of injury
Previous injury

▶ 2. INSPECTION

Girth measurements

Anterior Structures
Alignment of patella
Patellar tendon
Quadriceps muscle group
Alignment of the femur on the tibia
Tibial tuberosity

Medial Structures
Oblique fibers of vastus medialis

Lateral Structures
Fibular head
Posterior tibial sag
Hyperextension

Posterior Structures
Hamstring group
Popliteal fossa

▶ 3. PALPATION

Anterior Structures
Patella
Patellar tendon

Tibial tuberosity
Quadriceps muscle group
Sartorius

Medial Structures
Joint line/meniscus
Medial collateral ligament
Medial femoral condyle and epi-
    condyle
Medial tibial plateau
Pes anserine tendon and bursa
Semitendinosus tendon
Gracilis

Lateral Structures
Joint line/meniscus
Fibular head
Lateral collateral ligament
Popliteus tendon
Biceps femoris
Iliotibial band

Posterior Structures
Popliteal fossa
Hamstring muscle group

**Determination of Intracapsular
    Versus Extracapsular Swelling**
Sweep test
Ballotable patella

▶ 4. RANGE OF MOTION
        TESTS

Active Motion
Flexion and extension

93

Map

94 CHAPTER 6 The Knee

The Knee (Continued)

Internal and external rotation
(screw home mechanism)

Passive Motion
Flexion and extension

Resisted Motion
Flexion and extension
Isolating the sartorius

▶ **5. LIGAMENTOUS TESTS**

ACL Instability
Anterior drawer test
Lachman's test
Modified Lachman's test

PCL Instability
Posterior drawer test
Godfrey's test

MCL Instability
Valgus stress test

LCL Instability
Varus stress test

**Proximal Tibiofibular
   Syndesmosis**
Tibiofibular translation test

▶ **6. NEUROLOGICAL TESTS**

Peroneal nerve
Femoral nerve
Sciatic nerve
Lumbar nerve roots
Sacral nerve roots

▶ **7. SPECIAL TESTS**

Rotary Knee Instabilities
Slocum drawer
Crossover test
Lateral pivot shift
Slocum ALRI
FRD test

Meniscal Tears
McMurray's test
Apley's compression
Apley's distraction

ITB Friction Syndrome
Noble's compression test
Ober's test

ALRI = anterolateral rotatory instability; FRD = flexion–rotation drawer; IT = iliotibial; LCL = lateral collateral ligament; MCL = medial collateral ligament; PCL = posterior cruciate ligament.

Knee

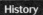

History

Table 6-1	Possible Trauma Based on the Location of Pain			
	Location of Pain			
	Lateral	Anterior	Medial	Posterior
Soft tissue	LCL sprain	ACL sprain (emanating from "inside" the knee)	MCL sprain	PCL sprain
	Lateral joint capsule sprain	Patellar tendinitis	Medial joint capsule sprain	Posterior capsule sprain
	Superior tibiofibular syndesmosis sprain	Patellar tendon rupture (partial or complete)	Medial patellar retinaculum irritation	Gastrocnemius strain
	Lateral patellar retinaculum irritation	Patellar bursitis	Pes anserine bursitis or tendinitis	Hamstring strain
	Biceps femoris strain	Patellar maltracking—chondromalacia	Semitendinosus strain	Popliteus tendinitis
	Biceps femoris tendinitis	Quadriceps contusion	Semitendinosus tendinitis	Popliteal cyst
	Popliteal tendinitis	Fat pad irritation	Semimembranosus strain	
	IT band friction syndrome	Quadriceps tendon rupture	Semimembranosus tendinitis	
	Lateral meniscus tear		Medial meniscus tear	
Bony	Fibular head fracture	Patellar fracture	Osteochondral fracture	
	Osteochondral fracture	Tibial plateau fracture	Osteochondritis dissecans	
	Osteochondritis dissecans	Sinding-Johansen-Larsen disease	Medial femoral condyle contusion	
	Lateral femoral condyle contusion	Osgood-Schlatter disease (in adolescents)	Medial tibial plateau contusion	
	Lateral tibial plateau contusion	Patellar dislocation or subluxation		
		Chondromalacia		

ACL = anterior cruciate ligament; IT = iliotibial; LCL = lateral collateral ligament; MCL = medial collateral ligament; PCL = posterior cruciate ligament.

Knee

Table 6–2 Mechanism of Knee Injuries and the Resultant Soft Tissue Damage

Force Placed on the Knee	Tensile Forces	Compressive Forces
Valgus	Medial structures: MCL, medial joint capsule, pes anserine muscle group, medial meniscus	Lateral meniscus
Varus	Lateral structures: LCL, lateral joint capsule, IT band, biceps femoris	Medial meniscus
Anterior tibial displacement	ACL, IT band, LCL, MCL medial and lateral joint capsules	Posterior portion of the medial and lateral meniscus
Posterior tibial displacement	PCL, popliteus, medial and lateral joint capsules	Anterior portion of the medial and lateral meniscus
Internal tibial rotation	ACL, anterolateral joint capsule, posteromedial joint capsule, posterolateral joint capsule, LCL	Anterior horn of the medial meniscus Posterior horn of the lateral meniscus
External tibial rotation	Posterolateral joint capsule, MCL, PCL, LCL, ACL	Anterior horn of the lateral meniscus Posterior horn of the lateral meniscus
Hyperextension	ACL, posterior joint capsule, PCL	Anterior portion of the medial and lateral meniscus
Hyperflexion	ACL, PCL	Posterior portion of the medial and lateral meniscus

ACL = anterior cruciate ligament; IT = iliotibial; LCL = lateral collateral ligament; MCL = medial collateral ligament; PCL = posterior cruciate ligament.

Knee

Inspection

Tibiofemoral Alignment

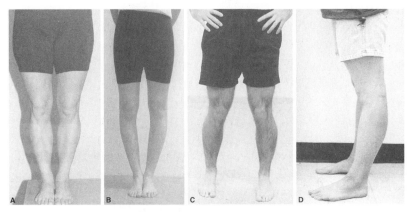

Figure 6–1 Alignment of the tibia on the femur. **(A)** Normal alignment, **(B)** genu varum (bow legs), **(C)** genu valgum (knockknees), and **(D)** genu recurvatum (hyperextension).

Girth Measurement

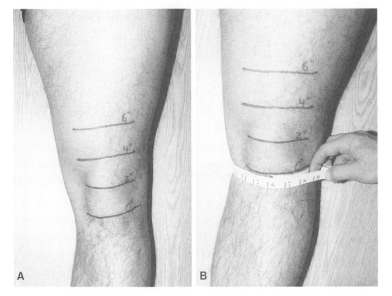

Knee

Figure 6–2 Girth measurements of the knee. Measurements are taken over the joint line (0 inches) to measure for swelling. Measurements are then taken at 2-inch increments around the thigh to determine the presence of atrophy (1-inch increments are used for smaller patients). These findings are then compared with the opposite extremity.

PALPATION

Palpation of the Anterior Structures

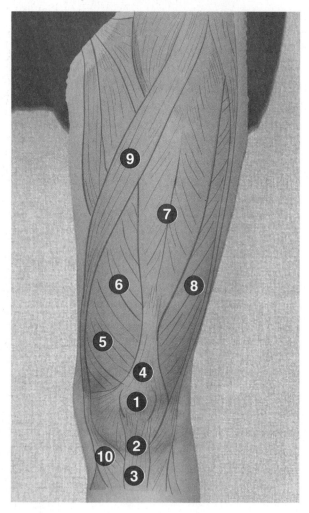

ANTERIOR KNEE

1 Patella
2 Patellar tendon
3 Tibial tuberosity
4 Quadriceps tendon
Quadriceps muscle group:
5 Vastus medialis oblique

6 Vastus medialis
7 Rectus femoris
8 Vastus lateralis
   (note: the vastus intermedius is not directly palpable)
9 Sartorius

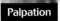

Palpation of the Medial Structures

![Illustration of the medial structures of the knee with numbered labels 1–7]

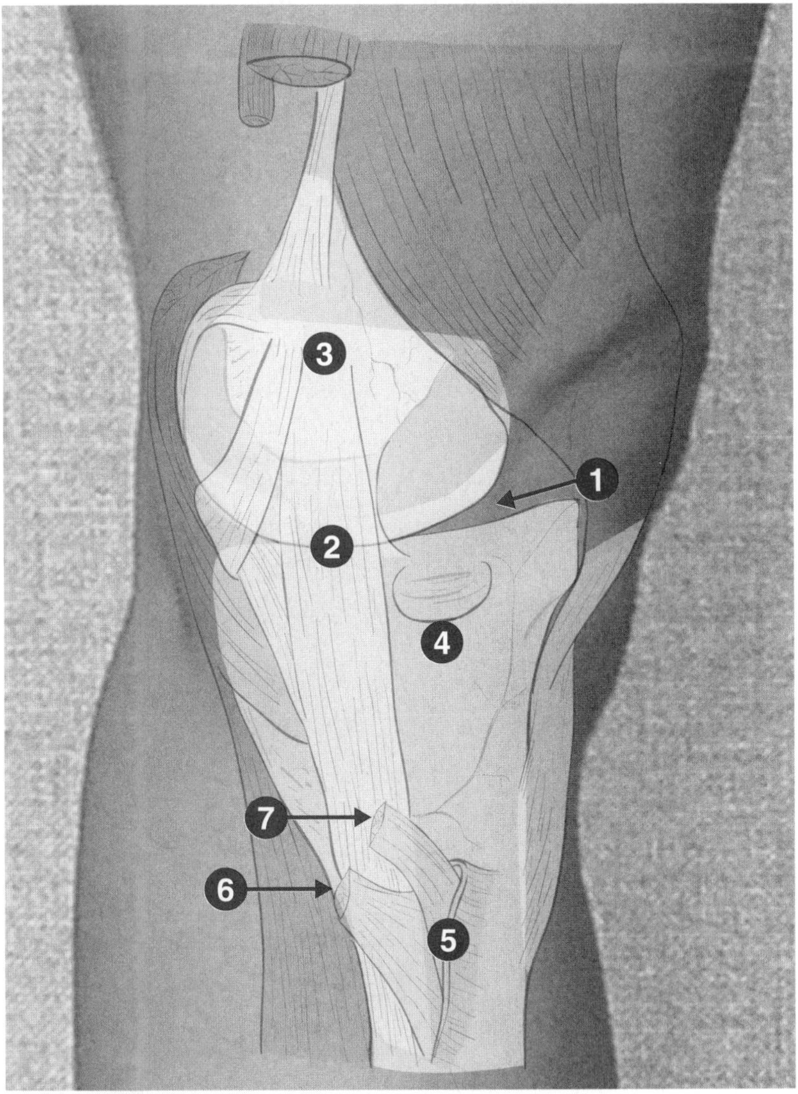

MEDIAL STRUCTURES

1 Medial meniscus and joint line
2 Medial collateral ligament
3 Medial femoral condyle and epicondyle

4 Medial tibial plateau
5 Pes anserine tendon and bursa
6 Semitendinosus tendon
7 Gracilis

Palpation of the Lateral Structures

Knee

LATERAL STRUCTURES

1 Joint line
2 Fibular head
3 Lateral collateral ligament
4 Popliteus
5 Biceps femoris
6 Iliotibial band

Palpation of the Posterior Structures

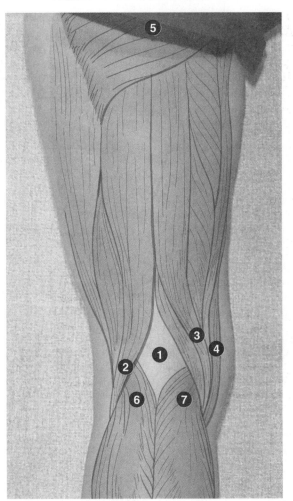

Knee

POSTERIOR STRUCTURES

1   Popliteal fossa
Hamstring muscle group:
2   Biceps femoris
3   Semimembranosus
4   Semitendinosus
6   Lateral head of the gastrocnemius
7   Medial head of the gastrocnemius

Range of Motion Testing

Box 6–1 Goniometry: Knee

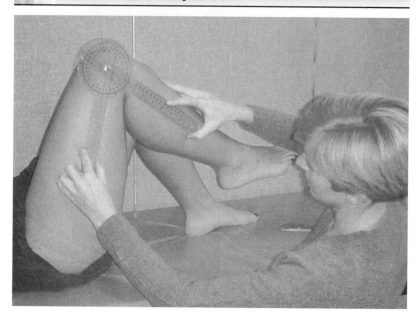

Knee

PATIENT POSITION	Lying supine. Knee flexion and extension may also be measured with the patient supine and a bolster placed under the distal femur.

GONIOMETER ALIGNMENT

FULCRUM	Centered over the lateral femoral epicondyle
STATIONARY ARM	Centered over the midline of the femur, aligned with the greater trochanter
MOVEMENT ARM	Centered over the midline of the fibula, aligned with the lateral malleolus

Table 6–3 Knee–Capsular Patterns and End-Feels

Capsular Pattern: Flexion, extension

Extension	Firm–Stretch of the posterior capsule; posterior capsule; ACL; PCL
Flexion	Soft–Soft tissue approximation between the triceps surae and the hamstrings
	Firm–Stretch of the rectus femoris
Internal tibial rotation	Firm–Stretch of the capsule; MCL; LCL; IT band
External tibial rotation	Firm–Stretch of the capsule; MCL; LCL; Pes anserine

ACL = anterior cruciate ligament; PCL = posterior cruciate ligament; MCL = medial collateral ligament; LCL = lateral collateral ligament; IT = iliotibial.

Knee Range of Motion: Flexion and Extension

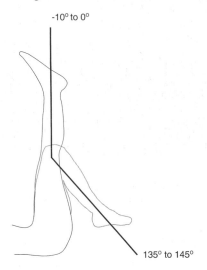

-10° to 0°

135° to 145°

Knee

Figure 6–3 Range of motion for flexion and extension of the knee.

Box 6–2 Resisted Knee Range of Motion

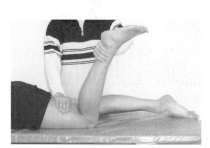
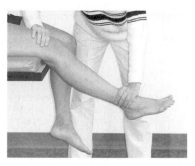

	Flexion	**Extension**
STARTING POSITION	The patient is prone and the knee is extended	The patient is seated with the knee flexed
STABILIZATION	Distal hamstrings	Distal quadriceps
RESISTANCE	Over the Achilles tendon	Proximal to the talocrural joint
MODIFICATION	Isometric break tests may be applied when the knee is flexed to 10°, 45°, and 90° unless this protocol is contraindicated by the patient's postoperative condition or other clinical findings.	Isometric break tests may be applied with the knee flexed to 15°, 45°, 90°, and 120° unless this protocol is contraindicated by the patient's postoperative condition or other clinical findings.
MUSCLES TESTED	Semimembranosus, semitendinosus, biceps femoris, sartorius, gastrocnemius, gracilis, popliteus	Rectus femoris, vastus lateralis, vastus intermedius, vastus medialis

Knee

Box 6–2 Resisted Knee Range of Motion (Continued)

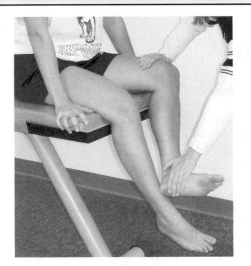

Isolating the Sartorius

STARTING POSITION	The heel of the leg being tested is positioned over the anterior talocrural joint with the patient sitting over the edge of the table.
RESISTANCE	Grasping the distal lower leg and over the distal quadriceps muscle.
MOTION	The patient attempts to slide the heel up the opposite tibia while resisting hip flexion, knee flexion, and femoral external rotation.

Knee

Tests for Joint Stability

Box 6–3   Anterior Drawer Test for Anterior Cruciate Ligament Laxity

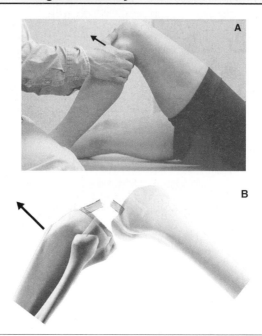

The anterior drawer test for anterior cruciate laxity **(A)**. Schematic representation of tibial displacement in a positive test **(B)**.

PATIENT POSITION	Lying supine Hip flexed to 45° and the knee to 90°
POSITION OF EXAMINER	Sitting on the examination table in front of the involved knee, grasping the tibia just below the joint line of the knee. The thumbs are placed along the joint line on either side of the patellar tendon. The index fingers are used to palpate the hamstring tendons to ensure that they are relaxed.
EVALUATIVE PROCEDURE	The tibia is drawn anteriorly.
POSITIVE TEST	An increased amount of anterior tibial translation compared with the opposite (uninvolved) limb or the lack of a firm end-point
IMPLICATIONS	A sprain of the anteromedial bundle of the ACL or a complete tear of the ACL
COMMENTS	The hamstring muscle group must be relaxed to ensure proper test results.

ACL = anterior cruciate ligament.

Knee

Box 6-4 Lachman's Test for Anterior Cruciate Ligament Laxity

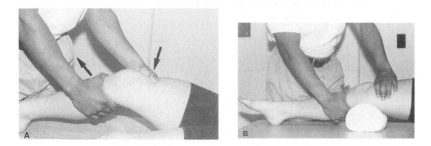

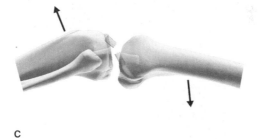

The Lachman test **(A)** and modification of the Lachman test **(B)**. Schematic representation of tibiofemoral translation in the presence of ACL deficiency **(C)**.

Knee

PATIENT POSITION	Lying supine The knee passively flexed to 20° to 25°
POSITION OF EXAMINER	One hand grasps the tibia around the level of the tibial tuberosity, and the other hand grasps the femur just above the level of the condyles.
EVALUATIVE PROCEDURE	While the examiner supports the weight of the leg and the knee is flexed to 20°, the tibia is drawn anteriorly while a posterior pressure is applied to stabilize the femur.
POSITIVE TEST	An increased amount of anterior tibial translation compared with the opposite (uninvolved) limb or the lack of a firm end-point
IMPLICATIONS	Sprain of the ACL
MODIFICATION	As shown in B above, the femur may be stabilized by placing a rolled towel beneath the knee to assist in stabilizing the femur.
COMMENTS	See Box 6-5, Alternate Lachman's Test

ACL = anterior cruciate ligament.

Box 6–5 Alternate Lachman's Test

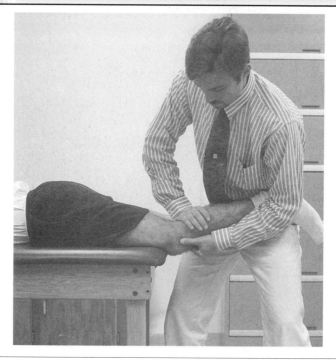

Alternate Lachman's test to differentiate between anterior tibial glide caused by ACL versus PCL laxity.

PATIENT POSITION	Prone The knee passively flexed to 30°
POSITION OF EXAMINER	Positioned at the legs of the patient so that the examiner supports the ankle The examiner's hand palpates the anterior joint line on either side of the patellar tendon
EVALUATIVE PROCEDURE	A downward pressure placed on the proximal portion of the posterior tibia as the examiner notes any anterior tibial displacement.
POSITIVE TEST	Excessive anterior translation relative to the uninvolved knee indicates a sprain of the ACL.
IMPLICATIONS	Positive test results found in the anterior drawer and/or Lachman's test and in the alternate Lachman's test indicate a sprain of the ACL A positive anterior drawer test and/or Lachman's test result and a negative alternate Lachman's test result implicate a sprain in the PCL.

ACL = anterior cruciate ligament; PCL = posterior cruciate ligament.

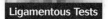

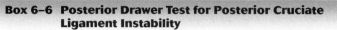

▓	**Box 6–6 Posterior Drawer Test for Posterior Cruciate Ligament Instability**

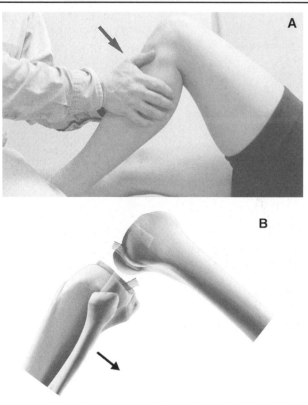

Knee

Posterior drawer test for PCL instability. **(A)** The tibia is moved posteriorly relative to the femur. **(B)** Translation of the tibia on the femur in the presence of a PCL tear.

PATIENT POSITION	Lying supine The hip flexed to 45° and the knee flexed to 90°
POSITION OF EXAMINER	Sitting on the examination table in front of the involved knee The patient's tibia stabilized in the neutral position
EVALUATIVE PROCEDURE	The examiner grasps the tibia just below the joint line of the knee with the fingers placed along the joint line on either side of the patellar tendon. The proximal tibia is pushed posteriorly.
POSITIVE TEST	An increased amount of posterior tibial translation compared with the opposite (uninvolved) limb or the lack of a firm end-point
IMPLICATIONS	A sprain of the PCL

PCL = posterior cruciate ligament.

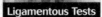

Box 6–7 Godfrey's Test for Posterior Cruciate Ligament Instability

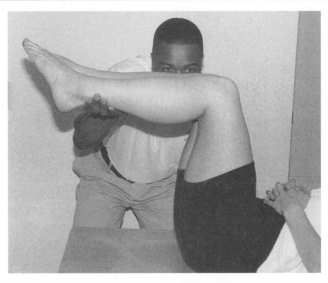

Godfrey's test for PCL laxity. Note the downward displacement of the left (facing) tibia

PATIENT POSITION	Lying supine with the knees extended and legs together
POSITION OF EXAMINER	Standing next to the patient
EVALUATIVE PROCEDURE	Lift the patient's lower legs and hold them parallel to the table so that the knees are flexed to 90°. Observe the level of the tibial tuberosities.
POSITIVE TEST	A unilateral posterior (downward) displacement of the tibial tuberosity
IMPLICATIONS	A sprain of the PCL
COMMENTS	The lower leg must be stabilized as distally as possible; supporting the tibia proximally prevents it from sagging posteriorly. An assistant may be used to hold the distal legs.

PCL = posterior cruciate ligament.

Knee

Box 6-8   Valgus Stress Test for Medial Collateral Ligament Instability

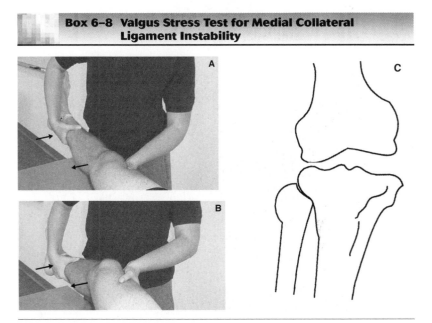

Valgus stress test **(A)** in full extension to determine the integrity of medial capsular restraints, **(B)** with the knee flexed to 25° to isolate the MCL, and schematic representation of the opening of the medial joint line **(C)**.

PATIENT POSITION	Lying supine with the involved leg close to the edge of the table
POSITION OF EXAMINER	Standing lateral to the involved limb One hand supports the medial portion of the distal tibia while the other hand grasps the knee along the lateral joint line. To test the entire medial joint capsule, the knee is kept in complete extension. To isolate the MCL, the knee is flexed to 25°.
EVALUATIVE PROCEDURE	A medial (valgus) force is applied to the knee while the distal tibia is moved laterally.
POSITIVE TEST	Increased laxity, decreased quality of the end-point, and pain compared with the uninvolved limb
IMPLICATIONS	In complete extension: a sprain of the MCL, medial joint capsule, and possibly the cruciate ligaments In 25° flexion: a sprain of the MCL
MODIFICATION	To promote greater relaxation of the patient's musculature, the thigh may be left on the table with the knee flexed over the side.
COMMENTS	When testing the knee in full extension, it is recommended that the thigh be left on the table, preventing shortening of the hamstring muscle group. The apprehension test (see Chapter 7) should be performed before valgus stress testing in patients who have a history of patellar dislocations or subluxations.

MCL = medial collateral ligament.

Knee

Box 6–9 Varus Stress Test for Lateral Collateral Ligament Instability

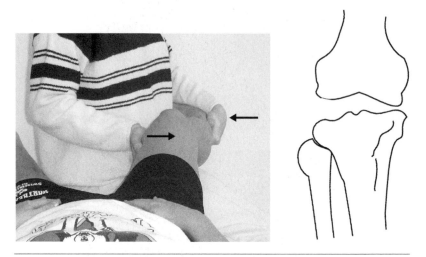

PATIENT POSITION	Lying supine with the involved leg close to the edge of the table
POSITION OF EXAMINER	Sitting on the table One hand supports the lateral portion of the distal tibia, while the other hand grasps the knee along the medial joint line. To test the entire lateral joint capsule, the knee is kept in complete extension. To isolate the LCL, the knee is flexed to 25°.
EVALUATIVE PROCEDURE	A lateral (varus) force is applied to the knee while the distal tibia is moved inward.
POSITIVE TEST	Increased laxity, decreased quality of the end-point, or pain compared with the uninvolved limb
IMPLICATIONS	In complete extension: a sprain of the LCL, lateral joint capsule, cruciate ligaments, and related structures, indicating possible rotatory instability of the joint In 25° of flexion: a sprain of the LCL
COMMENTS	When testing the knee in full extension, it is recommended that the thigh be left on the table, preventing shortening of the hamstring muscle group.

LCL = lateral collateral ligament.

Knee

Box 6–10 Tibiofibular Translation Test

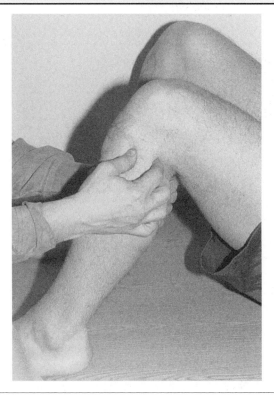

Knee

PATIENT POSITION	Lying supine with the knee passively flexed to approximately 90°
POSITION OF EXAMINER	Standing lateral to the involved side
EVALUATIVE PROCEDURE	One hand stabilizes the tibia while the other hand grasps the fibular head. While stabilizing the tibia, the examiner attempts to displace the fibular head anteriorly and then posteriorly.
POSITIVE TEST	Any perceived movement of the fibula on the tibia compared with the uninvolved side or pain elicited during the test
IMPLICATIONS	An anterior fibular shift indicates damage to the proximal posterior tibiofibular ligament; posterior displacement reflects instability of the anterior tibiofibular ligament of the proximal tibiofibular syndesmosis.

SPECIAL TESTS

Box 6-11 Sweep Test for Intracapsular Swelling

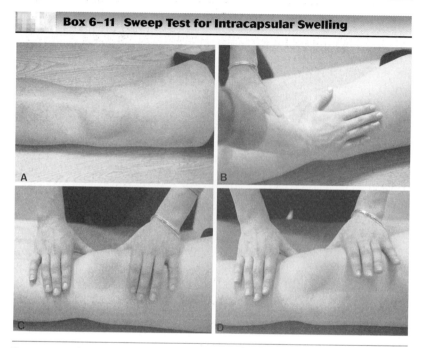

Sweep test to determine the presence of intracapsular swelling.

PATIENT POSITION	Lying supine with the knee extended
POSITION OF EXAMINER	Standing lateral to the patient
EVALUATIVE PROCEDURE	Assuming that the initial pocket of edema is on the medial side of the knee **(A)**: **(B)** The edema is stroked ("milked") proximally and laterally. **(C)** The normal contour of the knee is restored. **(D)** When pressure is applied on the lateral aspect of the knee, a fluid bulge immediately appears on the medial aspect.
POSITIVE TEST	Reformation of edema on the medial side of the knee when pressure is applied to the lateral aspect.
IMPLICATIONS	Swelling within the joint capsule, indicating possible anterior cruciate ligament trauma, osteochondral fracture, synovitis, meniscal lesion, or patellar dislocation.
MODIFICATION	If swelling is more prevalent on the lateral aspect of the knee, the steps are performed on the lateral side of the knee joint.

Knee

Box 6–12 Slocum's Drawer Test for Rotational Knee Instability

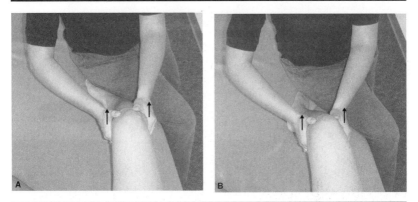

Slocum's drawer test with the tibia internally rotated to isolate the lateral capsular structures **(A)** and with the tibia externally rotated to isolate the medial capsule **(B)**.

PATIENT POSITION	Lying supine with the knee flexed to 90°
POSITION OF EXAMINER	Sitting on the patient's foot: **(A)** The tibia is internally rotated to 25° to test for anterolateral capsular instability. **(B)** The tibia is externally rotated to 15° to test for anteromedial capsular instability.
EVALUATIVE PROCEDURE	The tibia is drawn anteriorly.
POSITIVE TEST RESULT	An increased amount of anterior tibial translation compared with the opposite (uninvolved) limb or the lack of a firm end-point
IMPLICATIONS	**(A)** Test for anterolateral instability: damage to the ACL, anterolateral capsule, LCL, IT band, popliteus tendon, posterolateral capsule **(B)** Test for anteromedial instability: damage to the MCL, anteromedial capsule, ACL, posteromedial capsule

ACL = anterior cruciate ligament; IT = iliotibial; LCL = lateral collateral ligament; MCL = medial collateral ligament.

Knee

Knee

Box 6–13 Crossover Test for Rotational Knee Instability

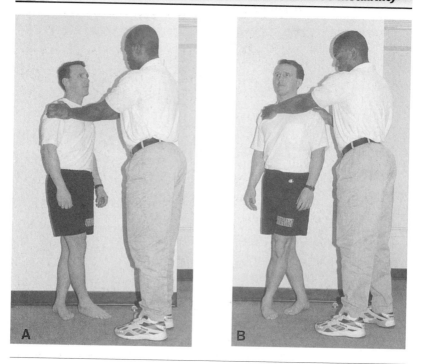

Crossover test: Stepping in front of the injured leg determines the presence of ALRI **(A)**. Stepping behind the injured leg determines AMRI **(B)**. Note that patient's left leg is being tested.

PATIENT POSITION	Standing with the weight on the involved limb
POSITION OF EXAMINER	Standing in front of the patient
EVALUATIVE PROCEDURE	**(A)** ALRI: The patient steps across and in front with the uninvolved leg, rotating the torso in the direction of movement. The weight-bearing foot remains fixated. **(B)** AMRI: The patient steps across and behind with the uninvolved leg rotating the torso in the direction of movement. The weight-bearing foot remains fixated.
POSITIVE TEST	Patient reports pain, instability, or apprehension
IMPLICATIONS	**(A)** ALRI: Instability of the lateral capsular restraints **(B)** AMRI: Instability of the medial capsular restraints

ALRI = anterolateral rotatory instability; AMRI = anteromedial rotatory instability.

Box 6–14 Lateral Pivot Shift Test for Anterolateral Knee Instability

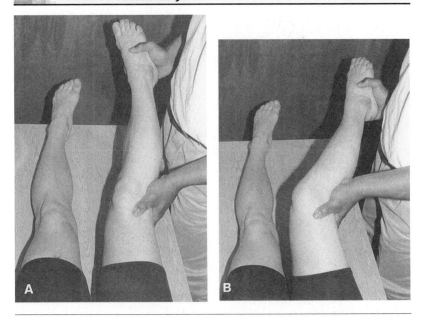

PATIENT POSITION	Lying supine with the hip passively flexed to 30°
POSITION OF EXAMINER	Standing lateral to the patient, the distal lower leg and/or ankle is grasped, maintaining 20° of internal tibial rotation. The knee is allowed to sag into complete extension (**A**). The opposite hand grasps the lateral portion of the leg at the level of the superior tibiofibular joint, increasing the force of internal rotation.
EVALUATIVE PROCEDURE	While maintaining internal rotation, a valgus force is applied to the knee while it is slowly flexed (**B**). To avoid masking any positive test results, the patient must remain relaxed throughout this test.
POSITIVE TEST	The tibia's position on the femur reduces as the leg is flexed in the range of 30° to 40°. During extension, the anterior subluxation is felt.
IMPLICATIONS	Tear of the ACL, posterolateral capsule, arcuate ligament complex, or the IT band
COMMENTS	Meniscal involvement may limit ROM to produce a false-negative test result. Muscle guarding can produce a false-negative result. This test is most reliable when performed by a physician while the patient is under anesthesia.

ACL = anterior cruciate ligament; IT = iliotibial; ROM = range of motion.

Box 6-15 Slocum's Anterolateral Rotatory Instability (ALRI) Test

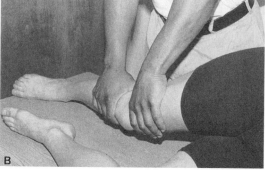

PATIENT POSITION	**(A)** Lying on the uninvolved side Uninvolved leg flexed at the hip and knee, moving it anterior to the involved extremity Involved hip externally rotated Involved leg extended with the medial aspect of the foot resting against the table to provide stability
POSITION OF EXAMINER	Standing behind the patient, grasping the knee on the distal aspect of the femur and the proximal fibula
EVALUATIVE PROCEDURE	A valgus force is placed on the knee, causing it to move into 30° to 50° of flexion **(B)**.
POSITIVE TEST	An appreciable "clunk" or instability as the lateral tibial plateau subluxates or pain or instability is reported
IMPLICATIONS	Tear of the ACL, LCL, anterolateral capsule, arcuate ligament complex, biceps femoris tendon and/or IT band.

ACL = anterior cruciate ligament; IT = iliotibial; LCL = lateral cruciate ligament.

Knee

Box 6-16 Flexion-Reduction Drawer Test for Anterolateral Rotatory Instability

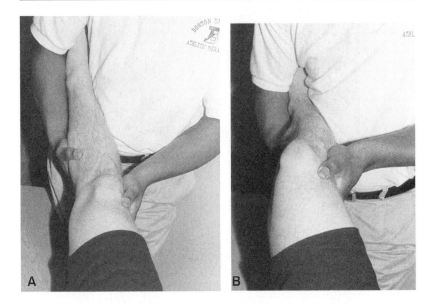

PATIENT POSITION	Lying supine
	The clinician lifts the calf and ankle so that the knee is flexed to approximately 25°.
	Heavier patients may require that the tibia be supported between the examiner's arm and torso.
POSITION OF EXAMINER	Standing lateral and distal to the involved knee
EVALUATIVE PROCEDURE	The tibia is depressed posteriorly to the femur.
	A valgus stress and axial compression along the tibial shaft are applied as the knee is slowly flexed.
POSITIVE TEST	The femur's relocating itself on the tibia by moving anteriorly and internally rotating on the tibia
IMPLICATIONS	Tear of the ACL, LCL, anterolateral capsule, arcuate ligament complex, biceps femoris tendon and/or IT band.

ACL = anterior cruciate ligament; IT = iliotibial; LCL = lateral cruciate ligament.

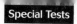

Box 6–17 External Rotation Test for Posterolateral Knee Instability

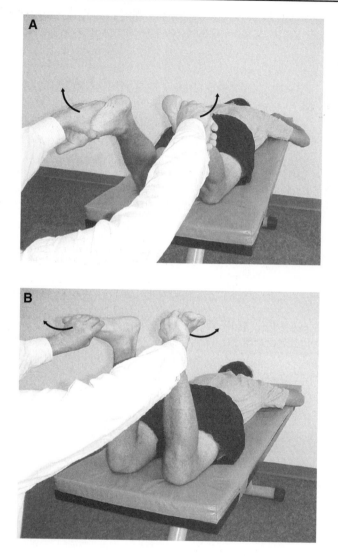

Box 6-17 External Rotation Test for Posterolateral Knee Instability (Continued)

The external rotation test for posterolateral knee instability at 30° of knee flexion **(A)** and at 90° of knee flexion **(B)**.

PATIENT POSITION	Prone or supine
POSITION OF EXAMINER	Standing at the patient's feet
EVALUATIVE PROCEDURE	The knee is flexed to 30° Using the medial border of the foot as a point of reference, the examiner forcefully externally rotates the patient's lower leg. The position of external rotation of the foot relative to the femur is assessed and compared with the opposite extremity. The knee is then flexed to 90° and the test repeated.
POSITIVE TEST	An increase of external rotation greater than 10° compared with the opposite side
IMPLICATIONS	Difference at 30° of knee flexion but not at 90°: injury isolated to the arcuate ligament complex and the posterolateral structures of the knee Difference at 30° and 90° of knee flexion: trauma to the PCL, posterolateral knee structures, and the arcuate ligament complex Difference at 90° of knee flexion but not at 30°: isolated PCL sprain
COMMENTS	This test can also be performed with the patient in the supine position. Normal variations for rotation are expected. The results of one extremity must be compared with those of the opposite leg.

PCL = posterior cruciate ligament.

Knee

Knee

Box 6–18 McMurray's Test for Meniscal Lesions

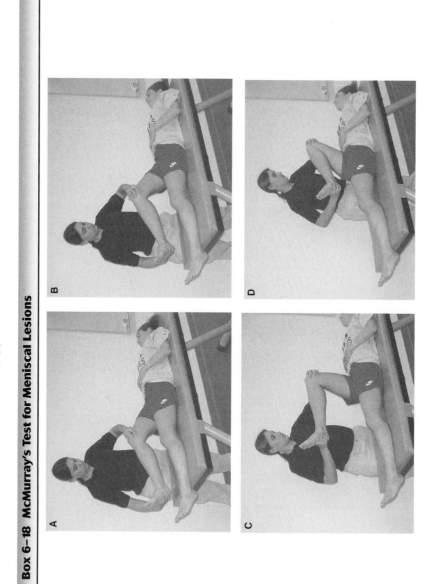

Box 6-18 McMurray's Test for Meniscal Lesions (Continued)

PATIENT POSITION	Lying supine
POSITION OF EXAMINER	Standing lateral and distal to the involved knee One hand supporting the lower leg while the thumb and index finger of the opposite hand positioned in the anteromedial and anterolateral joint line on either side of the patellar tendon (**A**).
EVALUATIVE PROCEDURE	(**B**) Pass one: With the tibia maintained in its neutral position, a valgus stress is applied while the knee is flexed through its available ROM. A varus stress is then applied as the knee is returned to full extension. (**C**) Pass two: The examiner internally rotates the tibia and applies a valgus stress while the knee is flexed through its available ROM. A varus stress is then applied as the knee is returned to full extension. (**D**) Pass three: With the tibia externally rotated, the examiner applies a valgus stress while the knee is flexed through its available ROM. A varus stress is then applied as the knee is returned to full extension.
POSITIVE TEST	A popping, clicking, or locking of the knee; pain emanating from the menisci; or a sensation similar to that experienced during ambulation
IMPLICATIONS	A meniscal tear on the side of the reported symptoms
COMMENTS	In acute injuries, the available ROM may not be sufficient to perform this test. Full flexion is required to isolate the posterior horns of the meniscus. Chondromalacia patellae or improper tracking of the patella may produce a click resembling that associated with a meniscal tear.

ROM = range of motion.

Knee

Box 6–19 Apley's Compression and Distraction Tests for Meniscal Lesions

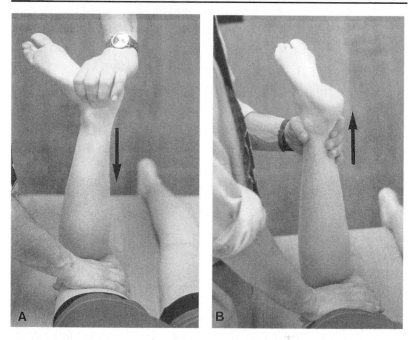

During the compression segment, pain may be caused by the menisci being caught between the tibia and femur **(A)**. During the distraction segment, the joint's ligaments are stressed **(B)**. Also, pain exhibited during compression should be reduced as the tibia is distracted from the femur.

PATIENT POSITION	Lying prone with knee flexed to 90°
POSITION OF EXAMINER	Standing lateral to the involved side
EVALUATIVE PROCEDURE	**(A)** Compression test: the clinician applies pressure to the plantar aspect of the heel, applying an axial load to the tibia while simultaneously internally and externally rotating the tibia. **(B)** Distraction test: the clinician grasps the lower leg and stabilizes the knee proximal to the femoral condyles. The tibia is distracted away from the femur while internally and externally rotating the tibia.
POSITIVE TEST	Pain experienced during compression that is reduced or eliminated during distraction
IMPLICATIONS	Meniscal tear
COMMENTS	Pain that is experienced only during distraction or during both compression and distraction may indicate trauma to the collateral ligaments, joint capsule, or cruciate ligaments.

Knee

Box 6–20 Wilson's Test for Osteochondral Defects of the Knee

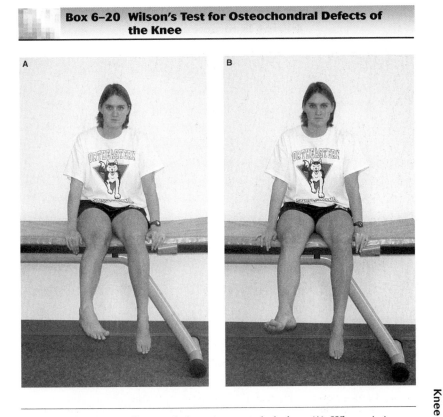

A   B

While the tibia is internally rotated, the patient extends the knee **(A)**. When pain is experienced, the patient externally rotates the tibia **(B)**. In the presence of some OCDs, pain is relieved during the external rotation.

PATIENT POSITION	Sitting with the knee flexed to 90°
POSITION OF EXAMINER	In front of the patient to observe any reactions secondary to pain
EVALUATIVE PROCEDURE	**(A)** The patient actively extends the knee while maintaining the tibia in internal rotation. The patient is told to stop the motion and hold the knee in the position in which pain is experienced. **(B)** If pain is experienced, the patient is instructed to externally rotate the tibia while the knee is held at its present point of flexion.
POSITIVE TEST	Pain experienced during extension with internal tibial rotation that is relieved by externally rotating the tibia
IMPLICATIONS	OCD or osteochondritis dissecans on the intercondylar area of the medial femoral condyle

OCD = osteochondral defect.

Knee

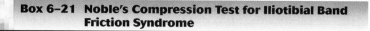

Box 6–21 Noble's Compression Test for Iliotibial Band Friction Syndrome

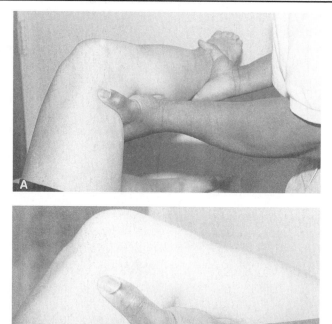

The examiner attempts to compress the distal portion of the IT band against the lateral femoral condyle during passive motion of the knee. In the presence of IT band inflammation, pain will be elicited.

PATIENT POSITION	Lying supine with the knee flexed
POSITION OF EXAMINER	Standing lateral to the side being tested The knee supported above the joint line with the thumb over or just superior to the lateral femoral condyle **(A)** The opposite hand controlling the lower leg
EVALUATIVE PROCEDURE	While applying pressure over the lateral femoral condyle, the knee is passively extended and flexed **(B)**.
POSITIVE TEST	Pain under the thumb, most commonly as the knee approaches 30°
IMPLICATIONS	Inflammation of the IT band, its associated bursa, or inflammation of the lateral femoral condyle

IT = iliotibial.

Knee

Box 6–22 Ober's Test for Iliotibial Band Tightness

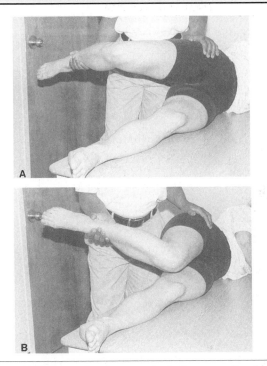

To eliminate false-positive test results, the tensor fasciae latae must first clear the greater trochanter. A positive test result occurs when the knee does not adduct past parallel.

PATIENT POSITION	Lying on the side opposite that being tested with the tested knee in flexion The opposite leg (i.e., the bottom leg) may be flexed to 90° at the knee and hip to stabilize the torso and pelvis.
POSITION OF EXAMINER	Standing behind the patient The leg grasped along the medial aspect of the proximal tibia
EVALUATIVE PROCEDURE	The examiner abducts and extends the hip to allow the tensor fasciae latae to clear the greater trochanter (**A**). The hip is then allowed to passively adduct to the table with the knee kept straight.
POSITIVE TEST	The leg is unable to adduct past parallel (**B**).
IMPLICATIONS	Tightness of the IT band, predisposing the individual to IT band friction syndrome and/or lateral patellar malalignment.
COMMENTS	With the involved knee flexed to 90°, the examiner should be aware that this position places tension on the femoral nerve (see Femoral Nerve Traction Test in Chapter 10) and on the medial structure of the knee. To avoid these complications, the Ober test may be performed with the knee in extension.

IT = iliotibial.

Neurological Testing

Neurological Symptoms in the Knee

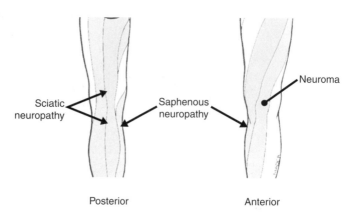

Posterior

Anterior

Figure 6–4 Local neuropathies of the knee. These findings should also be correlated with a lower quarter neurological screen.

The Patellofemoral Articulation

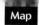
Map

Patellofemoral Joint (Continued)

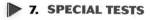

Femoral nerve
Sciatic nerve
Lumbar nerve roots
Sacral nerve roots

▶ **7. SPECIAL TESTS**

Patellar Dislocation
Apprehension test

Synovial Plica
Test for medial synovial plica
Stutter test

History

Table 7–1 Subjective Findings in the Differentiation of Meniscal and Patellar Pain

History	Meniscus	Patella
Onset	Usually acute twisting injury	Occasionally direct anterior knee blow but usually insidious related to overuse and training errors
Symptom site	Localized medial or lateral joint line	Diffuse, most commonly anterior
Locking	Frank transient locking episodes with the knee unable to fully terminally extend	Catching without locking, stiffness after immobility, but not true locking
Weight bearing	Pain sharp and simultaneous with loaded weight bearing	Pain possibly coming on during weight bearing but often continuing into the evening and night
Cutting sports	Pain with loaded twisting maneuvers	Some pain possible, but not sharp and clearly related to cutting
Squatting	Pain at full squat; inability to "duck walk"	Pain when extensors used to rise from a squat
Kneeling	Not painful because meniscus is not weight loaded	Pain from patellar compression
Jumping	Weight loaded without torque or twist tolerated	Extensors heavily stressed, causing pain on descent impact
Stairs or hills	Pain often going upstairs with loaded knee flexion, causing squatlike meniscal compression	More patellar loading and pain going downstairs because gravity-assisted impact increases patellofemoral stress
Sitting	No pain	Stiffness and pain from lack of the distraction-compression effect on abnormal articular cartilage

Patellofemoral

Inspection

Box 7-1   Patellar Position

Patella Alta	Patella Baja

Description

High-riding patellae; the camel sign may be present	Low-riding patellae

Potential causes

Abnormally long patellar tendon	Abnormally short patellar tendon Arthrofibrosis after surgery or injury

Consequences

Increased patellar glide, decreased quadriceps strength, increased patellofemoral compressive forces when the knee is flexed	Decreased patellar glide, decreased tibiofemoral range of motion, decreased quadriceps strength, increased patellofemoral compressive forces when the knee is flexed

Patellofemoral

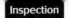
Box 7-1 **Patellar Position** (Continued)

Squinting Patellae	**"Frog Eyed" Patella**
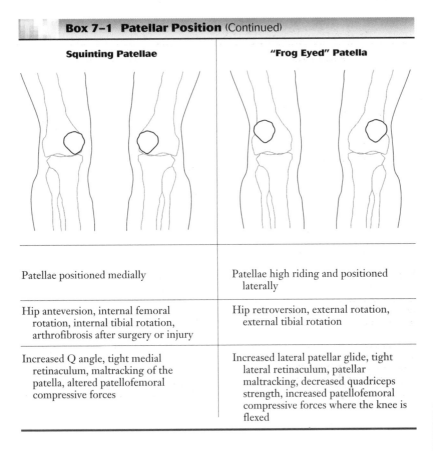	
Patellae positioned medially	Patellae high riding and positioned laterally
Hip anteversion, internal femoral rotation, internal tibial rotation, arthrofibrosis after surgery or injury	Hip retroversion, external rotation, external tibial rotation
Increased Q angle, tight medial retinaculum, maltracking of the patella, altered patellofemoral compressive forces	Increased lateral patellar glide, tight lateral retinaculum, patellar maltracking, decreased quadriceps strength, increased patellofemoral compressive forces where the knee is flexed

Patellofemoral

PALPATION

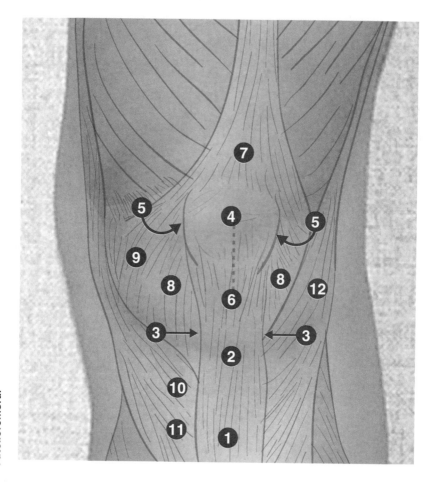

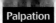
1 Tibial tuberosity
2 Patellar tendon and bursae
3 Fat pads
4 Patella and bursae
5 Patellar articulating surface
6 Femoral trochlea
7 Suprapatellar bursa
8 Retinaculum and capsular structures
9 Synovial plica
10 Pes anserine
11 Infrapatellar branch of the saphenous nerve
12 Iliotibial band

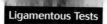

Ligamentous Testing

Box 7–2 Patellar Glide Tests

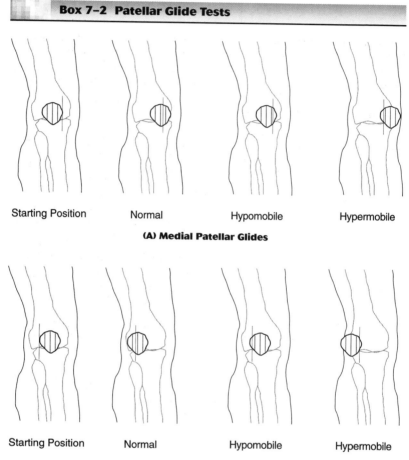

| Starting Position | Normal | Hypomobile | Hypermobile |

(A) Medial Patellar Glides

| Starting Position | Normal | Hypomobile | Hypermobile |

(B) Lateral Patellar Glides

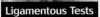

Box 7–2 Patellar Glide Tests (Continued)	

During medial **(A)** and lateral **(B)** patellar glide tests, the patella is viewed as having four quadrants. The amount of glide is based on the movement relative to the quadrants.

PATIENT POSITION	Supine with a bolster placed under the knee so that it is flexed to 30°
POSITION OF EXAMINER	Standing lateral to the patient
EVALUATIVE PROCEDURE	**(A)** Medial glide: Move the patella medially, placing stress on the lateral retinaculum and other soft tissue restraints. **(B)** Lateral glide: Move the patella laterally, placing stress on the medial retinaculum, VMO, and medial capsule.
POSITIVE TEST	Medial glide: The patella should glide one to two quadrants (approximately half its width) medially. Movement of less than one quadrant is hypomobile medial glide. Movement more than two quadrants is hypermobile medial glide. Lateral glide: Normal lateral motion is 0.5 to 2.0 quadrants of glide. Less than that is hypomobile lateral glide; greater than two quadrants is hypermobile lateral glide.
IMPLICATIONS	Medial glide: Hypomobile glide is the result of tightness of the lateral retinaculum or IT band. Hypermobile medial glide indicates laxity of the lateral restraints. Lateral glide: Hypomobile lateral glide is caused by tightness of the medial restraints. Laxity of the medial restraints results in hypermobile lateral glide, a predisposition to patellar dislocations.
COMMENT	The patient may be apprehensive during lateral glide tests, fearful that the motion could result in patellar dislocation.

IT = iliotibial; VMO = oblique fibers of the vastus medialis.

Patellofemoral

Box 7–3 Patellar Tilt Test

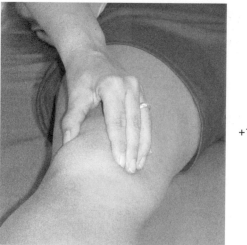

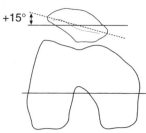

The patellar tilt test evaluates rotation of the patella around its midsagittal axis.

PATIENT POSITION	Supine with the knee extended and the femoral condyles parallel to the table
POSITION OF EXAMINER	Standing lateral to the patient
EVALUATIVE PROCEDURE	Grasp the patella with the forefinger and thumb, elevating the lateral border and depressing the medial border.
POSITIVE TEST RESULT	A normal result is the lateral border raising between 0° and 15°. More than 15° is a hypermobile lateral tilt; less than 0° is a hypomobile lateral tilt.
IMPLICATIONS	A tilt of less than 0° indicates tightness of the lateral restraints and often occurs in the presence of a hypomobile medial glide. A tilt of more than 15° may predispose the individual to anterior knee pain.

Patellofemoral

SPECIAL TESTS

Box 7–4   Q Angle Measurement with the Knee Extended

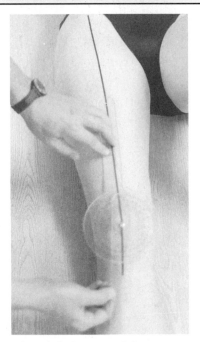

Measurement of the Q angle with the knee extended in a non–weight-bearing position; the anatomic landmarks of the ASIS, center of the patella, and the tibial tuberosity are used to align the goniometer

PATIENT POSITION	Lying supine with the knee fully extended
POSITION OF EXAMINER	Standing on the side of the limb to be measured
EVALUATIVE PROCEDURE	The examiner identifies and marks the ASIS, the midpoint of the patella, and the tibial tuberosity. A goniometer is placed so that the axis is located over the patellar midpoint, the center of the stationary arm is over the line from the ASIS to the patella, and the moving arm is placed over the line from the patella to the tibial tuberosity.
POSITIVE TEST	A Q angle greater than 13° in men or 18° in women
IMPLICATIONS	Increased lateral forces leading to a laterally tracking patella
MODIFICATION	These steps may be repeated with the patient standing. Re-measure the Q angle with the quadriceps isometrically contracted. Differences between the two measures may provide insight to patellar tracking deficits.

ASIS = anterior superior iliac spine.

Box 7–5   Q Angle Measurement with the Knee Flexed

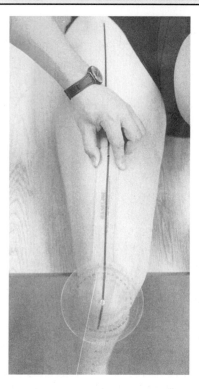

Measurement of the Q angle with the knee flexed to 90°; the anatomic landmarks of the ASIS, center of the patella, and the tibial tuberosity are used to align the goniometer.

PATIENT POSITION	Sitting with legs over the edge of the table with the knees flexed to 90°
POSITION OF EXAMINER	Standing on the side of the limb to be measured
EVALUATIVE PROCEDURE	The examiner identifies and marks the ASIS, the midpoint of the patella, and the tibial tuberosity. A goniometer is placed so that the axis is located over the patellar midpoint, the center of the stationary arm parallels the line from the ASIS to the patella, and the moving arm is placed over the line from the patella to the tibial tuberosity.
POSITIVE TEST	A Q angle greater than 8°
IMPLICATIONS	Increased lateral tracking during knee flexion, predisposing the patient to lateral patellar subluxations or dislocations

ASIS = anterior superior iliac spine.

Patellofemoral

Box 7-6 Clarke's Sign for Chondromalacia Patella

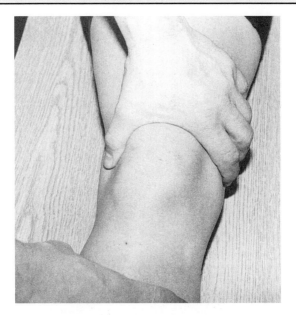

Clarke's sign for chondromalacia patella; this test elicits a great deal of pain and elicits a positive result in otherwise asymptomatic knees.

PATIENT POSITION	Lying supine with the knee extended
POSITION OF EXAMINER	Standing lateral to the limb being evaluated; one hand is placed proximal to the superior patellar pole, applying a gentle downward pressure
EVALUATIVE PROCEDURE	The patient is asked to contract the quadriceps muscle while pressure is maintained on the patella, pushing it into the femoral trochlea.
POSITIVE TEST	The patient experiences patellofemoral pain and the inability to hold the contraction.
IMPLICATIONS	Possibly chondromalacia patella The Clarke's sign is an unreliable test, producing false-positive results in otherwise asymptomatic knees.
MODIFICATION	The test may be performed with the knee flexed to various angles to assess different areas of patellofemoral contact.

Patellofemoral

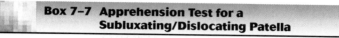

Box 7-7   Apprehension Test for a Subluxating/Dislocating Patella

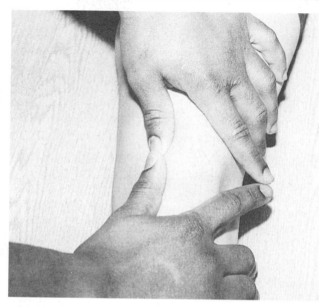

The apprehension test for patellar dislocation. The examiner glides the patella laterally. A positive test is indicated by the patient's contracting the muscle, describing pain, or otherwise showing apprehension (anticipation) of an impending dislocation.

PATIENT POSITION	Lying supine with the knee extended.
POSITION OF EXAMINER	Standing lateral to the involved side.
EVALUATIVE PROCEDURE	The examiner attempts to move the patella as far laterally as possible, taking care not to cause it to dislocate.
POSITIVE TEST	Forcible contraction of the quadriceps by the patient to guard against dislocation of the patella. The patient may also demonstrate apprehension verbally or through facial expression.
IMPLICATIONS	Laxity of the medial patellar retinaculum, predisposing the patient to patellar subluxations or dislocations.

Patellofemoral

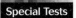

Box 7–8 Test for Medial Synovial Plica

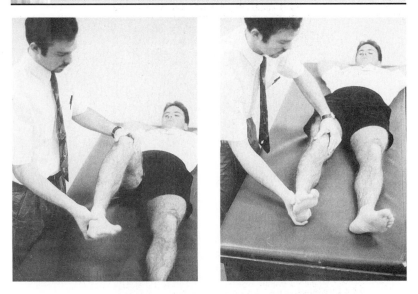

A positive test reproduces the patient's symptoms and the examiner may feel the plica as it crosses the medial femoral condyle.

PATIENT POSITION	Lying supine with the knee flexed or with the patient seated
POSITION OF EXAMINER	Standing on the side being tested
EVALUATIVE PROCEDURE	With the knee flexed to 90° and the tibia internally rotated, the examiner passively moves the patella medially while palpating the anteromedial capsule. The knee is then extended and flexed from 90° to 0° while the tibia is internally rotated.
POSITIVE TEST	Reproduction of the symptoms is described by the patient. The clinician may feel the plica as it crosses the medial femoral condyle, especially in the range of 60° to 45° of flexion.
IMPLICATIONS	Symptomatic medial synovial plica

Patellofemoral

Box 7–9 Stutter Test for a Medial Synovial Plica

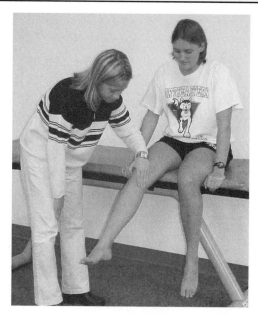

The examiner palpates the patella for irregular movement (stutter) as the patient extends the knee. When a plica snags against the medial femoral condyle, it may cause a momentary disruption in patellar motion.

PATIENT POSITION	Sitting with the knee flexed over the edge of the table
POSITION OF EXAMINER	Standing lateral to the involved side, lightly cupping one hand over the patella, being careful not to compress the articular surfaces
EVALUATIVE PROCEDURE	The patient slowly extends the knee.
POSITIVE TEST	Irregular motion or stuttering between 40° and 60° as the plica passes over the medial condyle
IMPLICATIONS	Medial synovial plica

8

The Pelvis and Thigh

EVALUATION MAP: Pelvis and Thigh

▶ 1. HISTORY
Location of symptoms
Onset
Training techniques
Mechanism of injury

▶ 2. INSPECTION

Hip Angulations
Angle of inclination
Angle of torsion

Medial Structures
Adductor group

Anterior Structures
Hip flexors

Lateral Structures
Iliac crest
Nélaton's line

Posterior Structures
Gluteus maximus
Posterior superior iliac spine
Median sacral crests

Leg Length Discrepancy
Functional leg length discrepancy
True leg length discrepancy
Apparent leg length discrepancy

▶ 3. PALPATION

Medial Structures
Pubic bone
Adductor muscle group

Anterior Structures
Anterior superior iliac spine
Anterior inferior iliac spine
Sartorius
Rectus femoris

Lateral Structures
Iliac crest
Greater trochanter
Gluteus medius
Tensor fasciae latae

Posterior Structures
Median sacral crests
Posterior superior iliac spine
Ischial tuberosity
Gluteus maximus
Hamstring muscles
Ischial bursa
Sciatic nerve

▶ 4. RANGE OF MOTION TESTS

AROM
Flexion
Extension
Adduction
Abduction
Internal rotation
External rotation

PROM
Flexion
Extension
Adduction

Pelvis and Thigh (Continued)

Abduction
Internal rotation
External rotation

RROM
Flexion
  Iliopsoas
  Rectus femoris
  Sartorius
Extension
  Hamstrings
  Gluteus maximus
Adduction
Abduction
Internal and external rotation
Thomas test for tightness of the hip
  flexors
Trendelenburg's test

▶ **5. LIGAMENTOUS TESTS**

Capsular testing
Flexion

Extension
Internal rotation
External rotation

▶ **6. NEUROLOGICAL TESTS**

Sciatic nerve compression
Lower quarter screen

▶ **7. SPECIAL TESTS**

Muscle weakness or tightness
  Trendelenburg's test
  Thomas' test
Degenerative hip changes
  Hip scouring
Piriformis syndrome

AROM = active range of motion; PROM = passive range of motion; RROM = resisted range of motion.

History

Table 8-1 Possible Trauma Based on the Location of Pain*

Location of Pain Medial	Anterior	Lateral	Posterior
Soft tissue Adductor strain Gracilis strain	Rectus femoris strain Iliopsoas strain Sartorius strain Symphysis pubis sprain Rectus femoris or iliopsoas tendinitis Iliofemoral bursitis Lymphatic edema	Trochanteric bursitis Gluteus medius strain Gluteus minimus strain	Ischial bursitis Hamstring strain Gluteus maximus strain
Bony Adductor avulsion fracture Stress fracture	Pubic bone fracture Arthritis	Iliac crest contusion Hip joint dysfunction	Sacroiliac pathology

* excluding gross injury.

PALPATION

Palpation of the Medial Structures

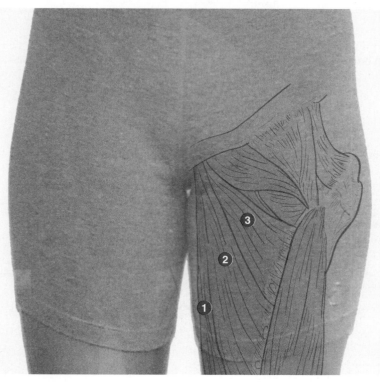

MEDIAL STRUCTURES

1 Adductor longus
2 Adductor magnus
3 Adductor brevis

Palpation of the Anterior Structures

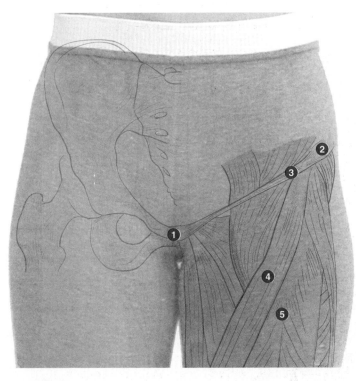

ANTERIOR STRUCTURES

1 Pubic bone
2 Anterior superior iliac spine
3 Anterior inferior iliac spine
4 Sartorius
5 Rectus femoris

Palpation of the Lateral Structures

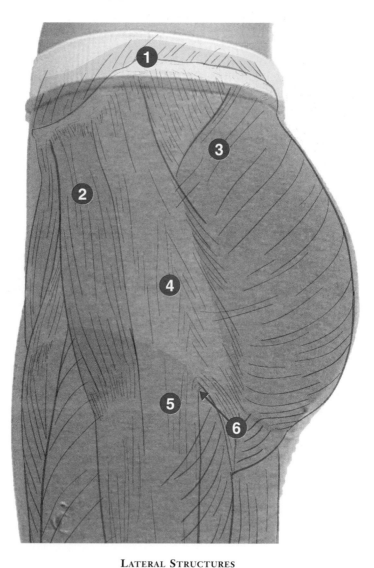

LATERAL STRUCTURES

1 Iliac crest	4 IT band
2 Tensor fasciae latae	5 Greater trochanter
3 Gluteus medius	6 Trochanteric bursa

Palpation of the Posterior Structures

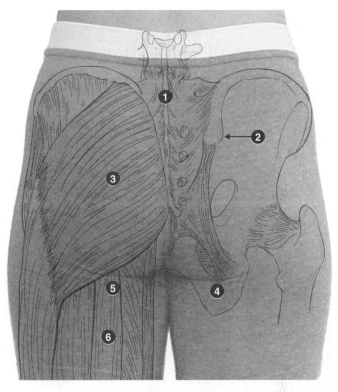

POSTERIOR STRUCTURES

1 Median sacral crests
2 Posterior superior iliac spine
3 Gluteus maximus

4 Ischial tuberosity and bursa
5 Sciatic nerve
6 Hamstring muscles

Pelvis and Thigh

Range of Motion Testing

Box 8-1 Goniometry: Hip

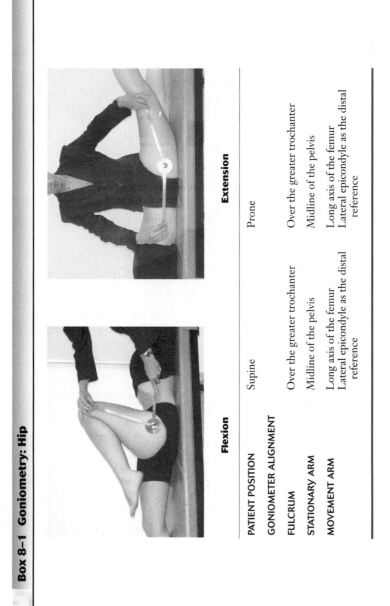

	Flexion	**Extension**
PATIENT POSITION	Supine	Prone
GONIOMETER ALIGNMENT		
FULCRUM	Over the greater trochanter	Over the greater trochanter
STATIONARY ARM	Midline of the pelvis	Midline of the pelvis
MOVEMENT ARM	Long axis of the femur Lateral epicondyle as the distal reference	Long axis of the femur Lateral epicondyle as the distal reference

Box 8-1 Goniometry: Hip (Continued)

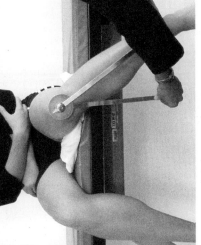

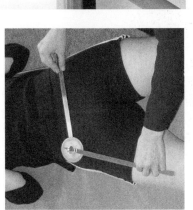

Abduction and Adduction	**Internal and External Rotation**
Supine; the opposite leg adducted during adduction	Seated
	Bolster placed under the distal femur to keep it parallel with the tabletop.
Over the ASIS	Center of the patella
The distal portion of the stationary arm is placed over the opposite ASIS.	Held perpendicular to the floor
Long axis of the femur	Long axis of the femur
Middle of the patella as the distal reference	The center of the talocrural joint as the distal reference

ASIS = anterior superior iliac spine.

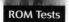

Table 8–2 Hip–Capsular Patterns and End-Feels

Capsular Pattern: Internal rotation, extension, abduction, flexion, external rotation

Extension	Firm–Soft tissue stretch of the anterior joint capsule; ischiofemoral 1.; pubofemoral 1.
Flexion	Soft–Contact between the anterior thigh and lower abdomen
	Firm–Stretch of the hamstring muscle group
Abduction	Firm–Stretch of the medial joint capsule; pubofemoral 1.; adductor muscle group; gracilis; pectineus
Adduction	Firm–Stretch of the lateral joint capsule; iliofemoral 1.; gluteus medius; gluteus minimus; tensor fasciae latae
Internal rotation	Firm–Tension in the posterior joint capsule; ischiofemoral 1.; small external hip rotator muscles
External rotation	Firm–Tension in the anterior joint capsule; iliofemoral 1.; pubofemoral 1.; gluteus medius; gluteus minimus; adductor magnus; adductor longus

Hip Range of Motion: Flexion and Extension

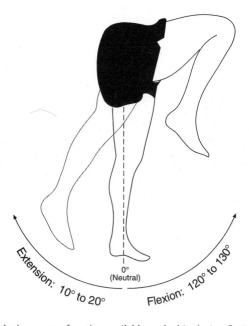

Figure 8–1 Active range of motion available to the hip during flexion and extension. The range for hip flexion is decreased when the knee is extended secondary to tightness of the hamstring muscles and is limited during extension when the knee is flexed because of tightness of the rectus femoris.

Hip Range of Motion: Abduction and Adduction

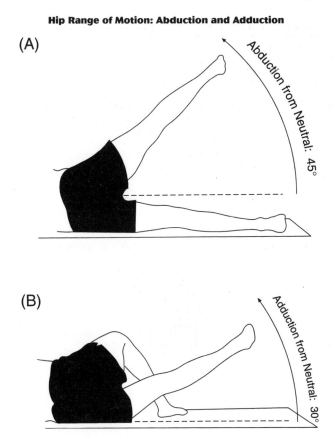

Figure 8–2 Active hip abduction **(A)** and adduction **(B)**.

Hip Range of Motion: Internal and External Rotation

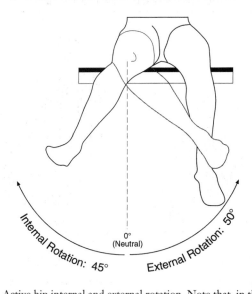

Figure 8–3 Active hip internal and external rotation. Note that, in the seated position, the lower leg moves in a direction opposite that of the femur (e.g., during internal femoral rotation the lower leg rotates outwardly).

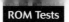
Box 8-2 Resisted Range of Motion: Hip

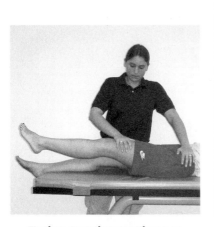

Flexion–Isolating the Iliopsoas

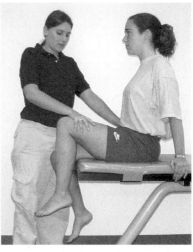

Flexion–Isolating the Rectus Femoris

STARTING POSITION	Supine or seated with the knee extended.	Seated with the knee flexed over the edge of the table.
STABILIZATION	Over the ASIS.	Pelvis stabilized.
RESISTANCE	Anterior aspect of the distal femur.	Anterior aspect of the distal femur.

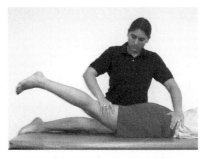

Extension–Isolating the Hamstrings

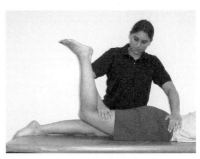

Extension–Isolating the Gluteus Maximus

STARTING POSITION	Prone with the knee extended.	Prone with the knee flexed to 90°.
STABILIZATION	Posterior pelvis.	Posterior pelvis.
RESISTANCE	Proximal to the popliteal fossa.	Posterior aspect of the distal femur.

Pelvis and Thigh

Box 8–3 Resisted Range of Motion: Hip

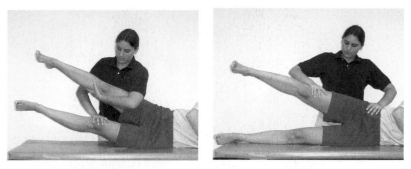

	Adduction	**Abduction**
STARTING POSITION	Sidelying on the side being tested with the knee extended. The opposite (nontested) leg supported by the examiner.	Sidelying on the opposite side being tested with the knee flexed slightly.
STABILIZATION	The pelvis and torso are actively stabilized by the patient.	The pelvis and torso are actively stabilized by the patient.
RESISTANCE	Over the medial femur, proximal to the knee	Over the lateral femoral condyle
MUSCLES TESTED	Adductor magnus, adductor longus, adductor brevis, gluteus maximus (lower fibers), gracilis, pectineus	Gluteus medius, gluteus maximus (upper fibers), gluteus minimus, sartorius

Box 8-3   Resisted Range of Motion: Hip (Continued)

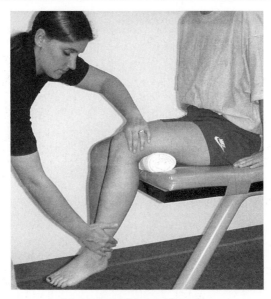

Internal and External Rotation

STARTING POSITION	Seated with the knees flexed over the edge of the table A bolster placed under the distal femur to keep it parallel with the tabletop
STABILIZATION	The patient's arms extended and supporting the torso on the table
RESISTANCE	On the side of the distal lower leg opposite the motion being tested
MUSCLES TESTED	Internal rotation (shown): Adductor longus, adductor magnus, adductor brevis, gluteus medius, gluteus minimus, semimembranosus, semitendinosus External rotation: Biceps femoris, gluteus maximus, piriformis, sartorius, gemellus inferior and superior, obturator internus and externus, quadratus femoris

ASIS = anterior superior iliac spine.

Pelvis and Thigh

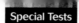

SPECIAL TESTS

Box 8–4 Clinical Determination of the Angle of Torsion

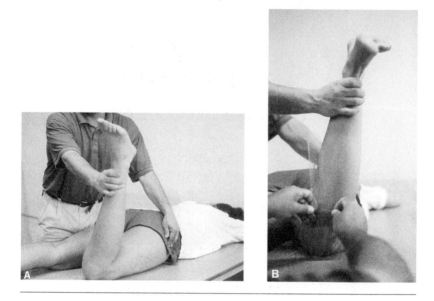

This procedure is most easily performed by two clinicians, one to manipulate the leg and the other to goniometrically measure the angle of the lower leg perpendicular to the table.

PATIENT POSITION	Prone with the knee of the leg being evaluated flexed to 90°
POSITION OF EXAMINER	The use of two examiners is recommended. Examiner 1: On the contralateral side to that being tested; one hand palpates the greater trochanter and the other hand manipulates the lower extremity. Examiner 2: Holding a goniometer distal to the flexed knee with the stationary arm perpendicular to the tabletop.
EVALUATIVE PROCEDURE	**(A)** Examiner 1 internally rotates the femur by moving the lower leg inward and outward until the greater trochanter is maximally prominent. This represents the point at which the femoral head is parallel with the tabletop. **(B)** Examiner 2 then measures the angle formed by the lower leg while the knee remains flexed to 90°.
POSITIVE TEST	Angles less than 15° represent femoral retroversion; angles greater than 15° represent anteversion.
IMPLICATIONS	As described in Positive Test above.

Box 8–5 Thomas Test for Hip Flexor Tightness

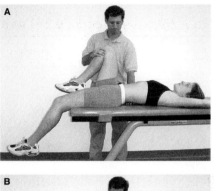

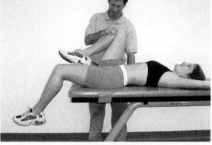

Thomas' test for hip flexor tightness. The patient's left (forward) leg is tested. **(A)** Tightness of the left rectus femoris muscle; **(B)** tightness of the left iliopsoas group.

PATIENT POSITION	Lying supine with the knees bent at the end of the table
POSITION OF EXAMINER	Standing beside the patient
EVALUATIVE PROCEDURE	The examiner places one hand between the lumbar lordotic curve and the tabletop. One leg is passively flexed to the patient's chest, allowing the knee to flex during the movement. The opposite leg (the leg being tested) rests flat on the table.
POSITIVE TEST	**(A)** The lower leg moves into extension. **(B)** The involved leg rises off the table.
IMPLICATIONS	**(A)** Tightness of the rectus femoris. **(B)** Tightness of the iliopsoas muscle group.
COMMENTS	The patient may passively flex the hip and knee by using the arms to pull the leg to the chest. The amount of lumbar flattening can be determined by placing a hand under the lumbar spine.

Pelvis and Thigh

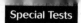

Box 8–6 Trendelenburg's Test for Gluteus Medius Weakness

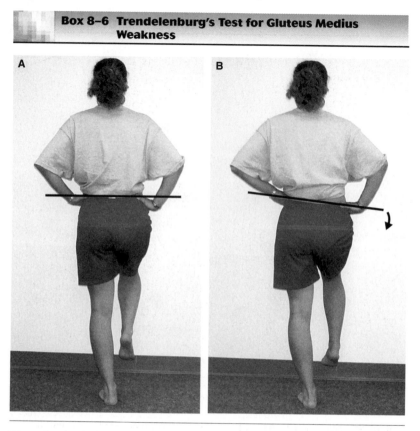

A   B

The patient is asked to stand on the affected leg (**A**). In the presence of gluteus medius weakness, the pelvis lowers on the opposite side of the affected leg (**B**).

PATIENT POSITION	Standing with the weight evenly distributed between both feet. The patient's shorts are lowered to the point at which the iliac crests or posterior superior iliac spines are visible.
POSITION OF EXAMINER	Standing, sitting, or kneeling behind the patient
EVALUATIVE PROCEDURE	The patient lifts the leg opposite the side being tested.
POSITIVE TEST	The pelvis lowers on the non–weight-bearing side.
IMPLICATIONS	Insufficiency of the gluteus medius to support the torso in an erect position, indicating weakness in the muscle or decreased innervation.

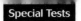
Box 8–7 Hip Scouring Test

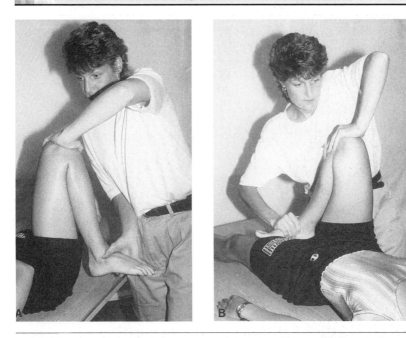

PATIENT POSITION	Supine
POSITION OF EXAMINER	At the side of the patient, fully flexing the patient's hip and knee
EVALUATIVE PROCEDURE	The examiner applies pressure downward along the shaft of the femur to compress the joint surfaces. The femur **(A)** internally and **(B)** externally rotated with the hip in multiple angles of flexion.
POSITIVE TEST	Pain described or symptoms in the hips reproduced
IMPLICATIONS	A possible defect in the articular cartilage of the femur or acetabulum (e.g., osteochondral defects, arthritis)
COMMENTS	This test may also produce pain in the presence of a labral tear.

Pelvis and Thigh

9

Evaluation of Gait

Monique Butcher, PhD, ATC

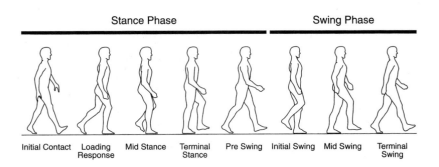

	Stance Phase				Swing Phase		
Initial Contact	Loading Response	Mid Stance	Terminal Stance	Pre Swing	Initial Swing	Mid Swing	Terminal Swing

Box 9-1 Stance Phase of Gait: Initial Contact

Initial Contact

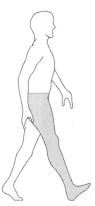

Weight-bearing surface

Subtalar joint
5° of supination

Talocrural joint
Neutral moving to 10° of dorsiflexion

Knee
0° of flexion: Tibia externally rotated

Hip
30° of flexion: Femur externally rotated

Muscle activity

Foot intrinsics
Isometric stabilization

Plantarflexors
Silent

Dorsiflexors
Eccentric

Quadriceps
Concentric

Hamstrings
Eccentric

Hip adductors
Eccentric

Gluteus maximus
Isometric to eccentric

Gluteus medius and minimus
Eccentric

Iliopsoas
Eccentric

Gait

Box 9–2 Stance Phase of Gait: Loading Response

Loading Response

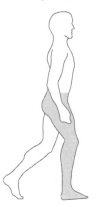

Weight-bearing surface

Subtalar joint
10° pronation

Talocrural joint
15° plantarflexion

Knee
15° flexion: Tibia internally rotates,
tibia begins to externally rotate as the
knee extends

Hip
30° flexion: Femur internally rotating to
neutral

Muscle activity

Foot intrinsics
Eccentric

Plantarflexors
Eccentric

Dorsiflexors
Eccentric

Quadriceps
Eccentric

Hamstrings
Isometric stabilization

Hip adductors
Eccentric

Gluteus maximus
Concentric

Gluteus medius and minimus
Isometric or concentric

Iliopsoas
Isometric stabilization

Box 9-3   Stance Phase of Gait: Midstance

Midstance

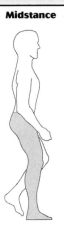

Weight-bearing surface

Subtalar joint
5° pronation, supinating toward neutral

Talocrural joint
0° to 5° dorsiflexion

Knee
15° flexion to 0°: Tibia externally
rotating

Hip
25° flexion to 0°: Femur internally
rotated

Muscle activity

Foot intrinsics
Concentric

Plantarflexors
Eccentric

Dorsiflexors
Concentric, but momentum can carry
the talocrural joint through its range
of motion.

Quadriceps
Silent

Hamstrings
Isometric

Hip adductors
Isometric

Gluteus maximus
Silent

Gluteus medius and minimus
Concentric

Iliopsoas
Eccentric

Box 9–4 Stance Phase of Gait: Terminal Stance

Terminal Stance

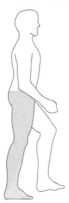

Weight-bearing surface

Subtalar joint
5° supination

Talocrural joint
5° to 10° dorsiflexion moving toward
  plantarflexion

Knee
5° flexion to 0°: Tibia externally rotates

Hip
0° to 10° extension: Femur externally
  rotates and adducts

Muscle activity

Foot intrinsics
Concentric

Plantarflexors
Eccentric to concentric

Dorsiflexors
Isometric

Quadriceps
Silent

Hamstrings
Concentric

Hip adductors
Isometric

Gluteus maximus
Isometric

Gluteus medius and minimus
Concentric

Iliopsoas
Eccentric

Box 9-5   Stance Phase of Gait: Preswing

Preswing

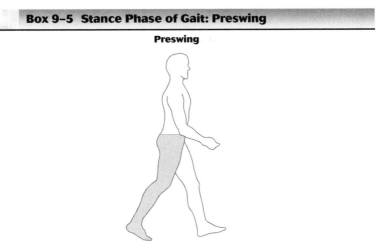

Weight-bearing surface

Subtalar joint
10° supination

Talocrural joint
0° to 20° plantarflexion

Knee
0° to 30° flexion: Tibia externally
  rotates

Hip
20° extension to 0° extension: Femur
  externally rotates with slight
  abduction

Muscle activity

Foot intrinsics
Concentric

Plantarflexors
Concentric

Dorsiflexors
Concentric to silent

Quadriceps
Eccentric to silent

Hamstrings
Concentric

Hip adductors
Eccentric to control the pelvis

Gluteus maximus
Isometric

Gluteus medius and minimus
Isometric

Iliopsoas
Concentric

Box 9–6 Swing Phase of Gait: Initial Swing

Initial Swing

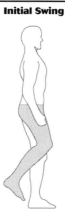

Limb position

Weight-bearing surface

Subtalar joint
Pronating

Talocrural joint
20° dorsiflexion

Knee
30° to 60° flexion: Tibia internally
rotates

Hip
0° to 20° flexion: Femur externally
rotates to neutral

Muscle activity

Foot intrinsics
Isometric stabilization

Plantarflexors
Concentric, reducing muscular activity

Dorsiflexors
Concentric until the foot is clear of the
ground, then isometric

Quadriceps
Concentric

Hamstrings
Concentric to eccentric

Hip adductors
Concentric

Gluteus maximus
Isometric

Gluteus medius and minimus
Isometric

Iliopsoas
Concentric

Gait

Box 9-7   Swing Phase of Gait: Midswing

Midswing

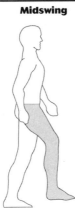

Limb position

Weight-bearing surface

Subtalar joint
Neutral

Talocrural joint
Neutral

Knee
30° to 0° flexion: Tibia externally
rotates

Hip
20° to 30° flexion: Femur externally
rotates

Muscle activity

Foot intrinsics
Isometric

Plantarflexors
Concentric

Dorsiflexors
Isometric

Quadriceps
Silent—Momentum carries the limb
through the ROM

Hamstrings
Eccentric

Hip adductors
Isometric

Gluteus maximus
Eccentric

Gluteus medius and minimus
Isometric

Iliopsoas
Concentric or silent

Gait

Box 9–8 Swing Phase of Gait: Terminal Swing

Terminal Swing

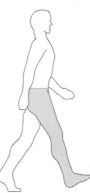

Limb position

Weight-bearing surface

Subtalar joint
5° supination

Talocrural joint
Neutral

Knee
0°: Tibia externally rotates

Hip
30° flexion: Femur externally rotates

Muscle activity

Foot intrinsics
Isometric stabilization

Plantarflexors
Isometric

Dorsiflexors
Isometric

Quadriceps
Concentric to stabilize the knee

Hamstrings
Eccentric

Hip adductors
Eccentric

Gluteus maximus
Eccentric

Gluteus medius and minimus
Isometric

Iliopsoas
Isometric

10

The Thoracic and Lumbar Spine

▶ 1. HISTORY

Location of the pain
Onset of the pain
Mechanism of injury
Consistency of the pain
Paresthesia
Activities or positions that alter the
  level of symptoms
Bowel or bladder signs
History of spinal injury

▶ 2. INSPECTION

General inspection
Frontal curvature
  Test for scoliosis
Sagittal curvature
  Lordotic and kyphotic curves
Observation of gait
Skin markings

Thoracic spine
Breathing patterns
Bilateral comparison of skinfolds

Lumbar spine
General movement and posture
Lordotic curve
Standing posture

▶ 3. PALPATION

Thoracic spine
Spinous processes
Supraspinous ligaments
Costovertebral junction
Trapezius
Scapular muscles
Paravertebral muscles

Lumbar spine
Spinous processes
Step-off deformity
Paravertebral muscles

Sacrum and pelvis
Median sacral crests
Iliac crests
Posterior superior iliac spine
Gluteals
Ischial tuberosity
Greater trochanter
Sacral nerve
Pubic symphysis

▶ 4. RANGE OF MOTION
  TESTS

AROM
Flexion
Extension

Map

174   CHAPTER 10   The Thoracic and Lumbar Spine

Lateral bending
Rotation

PROM
Flexion
Extension
Rotation
Side gliding

RROM
Flexion
Extension
Rotation

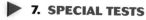

▶ 5. LIGAMENTOUS TESTS

Spring test for facet joint mobility

▶ 6. NEUROLOGICAL TESTS

Beevor's sign–thoracic nerve inhibition
Lower motor neuron lesions
  Upper quarter screen
  Lower quarter screen
Sciatic nerve compression

▶ 7. SPECIAL TESTS

Herniated disc
Valsalva test

Milgram test
Kernig's test/Brudzinski test
Well straight leg raising test
Quadrant test

Nerve Root Impingement
Quadrant test
Femoral nerve stretch test

Sciatic Nerve Involvement
Straight leg raise
Slump test
Tension sign/Bowstring test

Dural sheath irritation
Kernig's test/Brudzinski test

Spondylolysis/Spondylolisthesis
Single leg stance test

Sacroiliac Joint Dysfunction
Sacroiliac compression/distraction test
FABERE test
Gaenslen's test
Long sit test

Hoover test

AROM = active range of motion; PROM = passive range of motion; RROM = resisted range of motion.

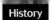

History

Table 10-1 Ramifications of Spinal Pain Exhibited During the Activities of Daily Living

Activity	Ramifications
Bending	Pain may be initially worsened with flexion exercises.
Sitting	Pain may be initially worsened with flexion exercises.
Rising from sitting	This motion causes changes in the interdiscal forces. Sharp pain suggests derangement of the disc.
Standing	The spine is placed in extension. Pain may be initially experienced with extension exercises.
Walking	The amount of spinal extension increases as the speed of gait increases.
Lying prone	The spine is placed in or near full extension.
Lying supine	When lying supine on a hard surface, the amount of extension is maintained. When lying on a soft surface, the spine falls into flexion.

PALPATION

Palpation of the Thoracic Spine

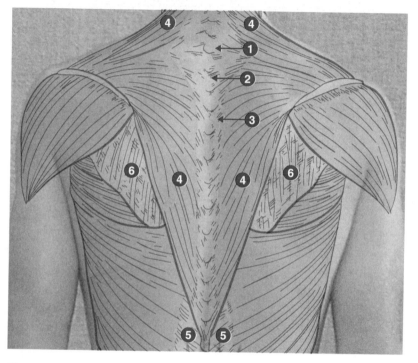

THORACIC SPINE

1 Spinous process
2 Supraspinous ligaments
3 Costeovertebral junction
4 Trapezius
5 Paravertebral muscles
6 Scapular muscles

Palpation of the Lumbar Spine

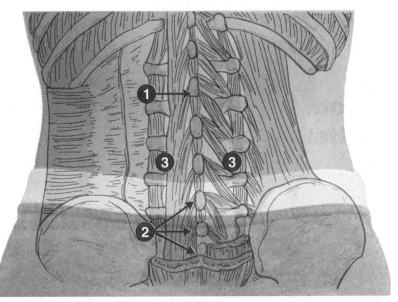

LUMBAR SPINE

1 Spinous processes
2 Step-off deformity of spinous process
3 Paravertebral muscles

Palpation of the Sacrum and Pelvis

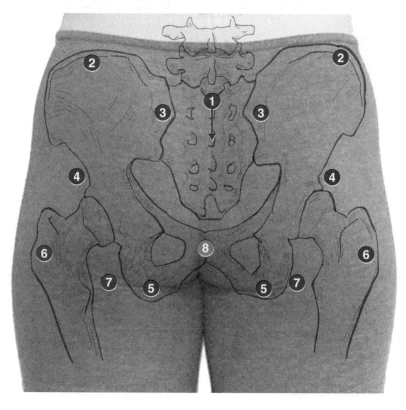

SACRUM AND PELVIS

1 Median sacral crests
2 Iliac crests
3 Posterior superior iliac spine
4 Gluteals
5 Ischial tuberosity
6 Greater trochanter
7 Sciatic nerve
8 Pubic symphysis

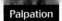
Table 10-2 Bony Landmarks During Palpation

Structure	Landmark
Cervical vertebral bodies	On the same level as the spinous processes
C1 transverse process	One finger's breadth inferior to the mastoid process
C3–C4 vertebrae	Posterior to the hyoid bone
C4–C5 vertebrae	Posterior to the thyroid cartilage
C6 vertebra	Posterior to the cricoid cartilage; moves during flexion and extension of the cervical spine
C7 vertebra	Prominent posterior spinous process
Thoracic spinal bodies	Underlying the spinous processes of the superior vertebra
T1 vertebra	Prominent protrusion inferior to the cervical spine; does not disappear during cervical extension
T2 vertebra	Posterior from the jugular notch of the sternum
T3 vertebra	Even with the medial border of the scapular spine
T7 vertebra	Even with the inferior angle of scapula
Lumbar spinal bodies	Upper portion of the spinous processes overlying the inferior half of the same vertebra
L3 vertebra	In normal body build, posterior from the umbilicus
L4 vertebra	Level with the iliac crest
L5 vertebra	Typically demarcated by bilateral dimples, but variable from person to person
S2	At the level of the posterior superior iliac spine

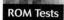
180   CHAPTER 10   The Thoracic and Lumbar Spine

Range of Motion Testing

Box 10–1   Goniometry: Trunk Range of Motion Testing

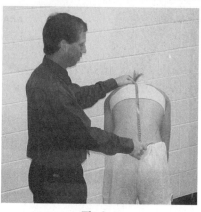

Flexion

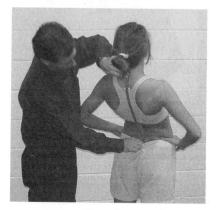

Extension

PATIENT POSITION	Standing with knees extended and the spine in the neutral position
PROCEDURE	The procedure is the same for flexion and extension.
INITIAL MEASUREMENT	Using a tape measure, the distance (in cm) between the C7 and S1 vertebrae is determined.
MOTION	The trunk is fully flexed or extended. Observe the pelvis for rotation that indicates compensation for spinal motion.
FINAL MEASUREMENT	The distance between the C7 and S1 vertebrae is determined. The difference between the initial and final measurement is calculated and the value recorded.

Box 10–1   Goniometry: Trunk Range of Motion Testing
(Continued)

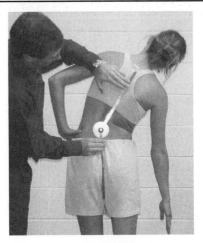

Lateral Bending

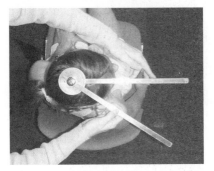

Rotation

	Lateral Bending	**Rotation**
PATIENT POSITION	Standing with the knees extended and the spine in the neutral position	Seated Feet placed firmly on the floor
GONIOMETER ALIGNMENT		
FULCRUM	Aligned over the S1 spinous process	Aligned over the center of the patient's head
STATIONARY ARM	Aligned over the median sacral crest	Parallel to the line formed by the iliac crests
MOVEMENT ARM	Aligned with the C7 vertebrae	Parallel to the line formed by the two acromion processes

Thorax and Lumbar

Box 10–2 Resisted Range of Motion for the Trunk

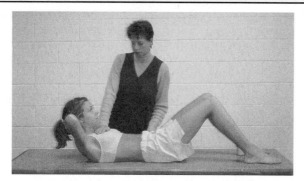

Flexion

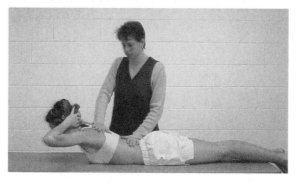

Extension

	Flexion	Extension
STARTING POSITION	Supine with the knees flexed and the feet flat on the table The patient's hands interlocked behind the head	Prone with the arms outstretched above the head, at the side, or interlocked behind the head
STABILIZATION	Pelvis	Lower lumbar region
RESISTANCE	Resistance is applied to the superior sternum as the patient lifts the scapulae off the table.	Resistance is applied to the upper thoracic spine as the patient lifts the head, chest, and arms off the table.
MUSCLES TESTED	Rectus abdominis, internal oblique, external oblique	Iliocostalis lumborum, iliocostalis thoracis, longissimus thoracis, spinalis thoracis, semispinalis thoracis, rotatores, latissimus dorsi

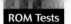

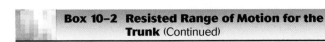

Box 10–2   Resisted Range of Motion for the Trunk (Continued)

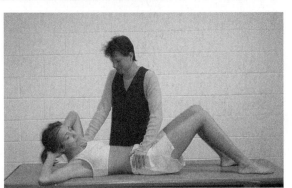

Rotation

STARTING POSITION	Supine. The patient's hands interlocked behind the head
STABILIZATION	Opposite ASIS
RESISTANCE	Resistance is applied over the anterior aspect of the shoulder as it is rotated off the table. This procedure is repeated for the opposite side.
MUSCLES TESTED	Internal oblique, external oblique (opposite side), rotatores, multifidi (opposite side)

ASIS = anterior superior iliac spine.

Ligamentous Testing

Box 10–3   Spring Test for Facet Joint Mobility

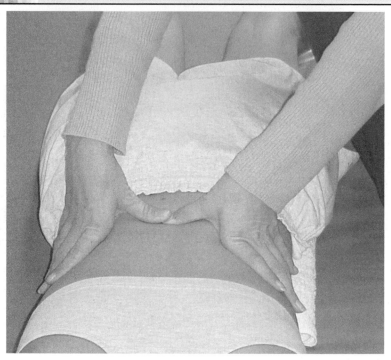

PATIENT POSITION	Prone
POSITION OF EXAMINER	Standing over the patient with the thumbs placed over the spinous process to be tested
EVALUATIVE PROCEDURE	The examiner carefully pushes the spinous process anteriorly, feeling for the springing of the vertebrae.
POSITIVE TEST	The vertebra does not move ("spring") or pain is elicited.
IMPLICATIONS	Hypomobility of the vertebrae, especially at the facet joints or a sprain

SPECIAL TESTS

Box 10–4   Test for Scoliosis

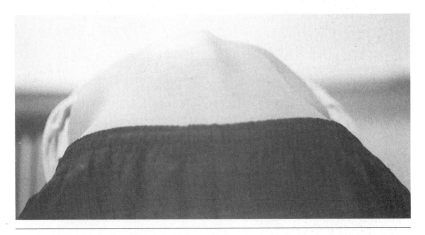

Posterior view of the spinal column while the patient flexes the spine; note the presence of a hump over the left thoracic spine, suggesting scoliosis.

PATIENT POSITION	Standing with hands held in front with the arms straight.
POSITION OF EXAMINER	Seated in front of or behind the patient.
EVALUATIVE PROCEDURE	The patient bends forward, sliding the hands down the front of each leg.
POSITIVE TEST	An asymmetrical hump is observed along the lateral aspect of the thoracolumbar spine and rib cage.
IMPLICATIONS	If scoliosis is present but disappears during flexion, then functional scoliosis is suggested. Scoliosis that is present while the patient is standing upright and while forwardly flexed indicates structural scoliosis.

Thorax and Lumbar

Box 10–5 Beevor's Sign for Thoracic Nerve Inhibition

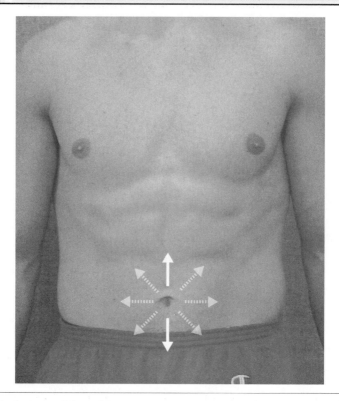

Lateral movement of the umbilicus can indicate inhibition of the nerves innervating the abdominal muscles.

PATIENT POSITION	Hook-lying
POSITION OF EXAMINER	At the side of the patient
EVALUATIVE PROCEDURE	The patient performs an abdominal curl (partial sit-up)
POSITIVE TEST	The umbilicus moves up, down, or to one side
IMPLICATION	Segmental involvement of the nerves innervating the rectus abdominis (T5 through T12); this should draw suspicion to the paraspinal muscles innervated by the same nerve roots.
COMMENT	Normally the umbilicus should not move at all during this test, but will move toward the stronger muscle group in the presence of pathology.

Box 10–6 Valsalva's Test

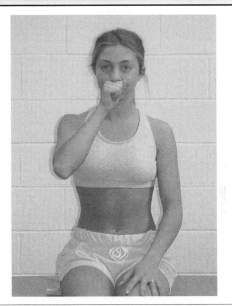

The Valsalva test attempts to increase intrathecal pressure, duplicating nerve-root pain that may be elicited while coughing or with bowel movements.

PATIENT POSITION	Sitting
POSITION OF EXAMINER	Standing within arms' reach in front of the patient
EVALUATIVE PROCEDURE	The patient takes and holds a deep breath while bearing down similar to performing a bowel movement.
POSITIVE TEST	Increased spinal or radicular pain
IMPLICATIONS	Increase in intrathecal pressure causes pain secondary to a space-occupying lesion such as a herniated disc, tumor, or osteophyte anywhere along the spinal column.
MODIFICATION	If the patient is embarrassed or apprehensive about simulating a bowel movement, he or she may be instructed to blow into a closed fist as if inflating a balloon.
COMMENTS	This can be performed for any level of the spine. The test increases intrathecal pressure, resulting in a slowing of the pulse, decreased venous return, and increased venous pressure, all of which may cause fainting.

Box 10–7 Milgram's Test

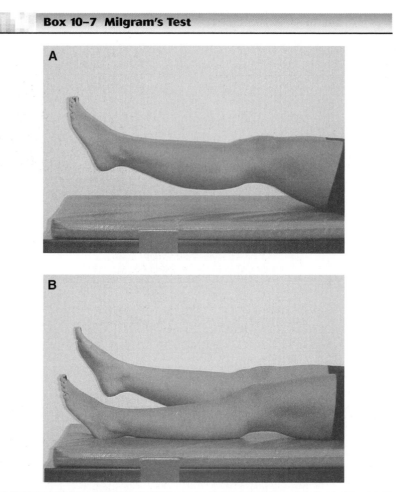

PATIENT POSITION	Supine
POSITION OF EXAMINER	At the feet of the patient
EVALUATIVE PROCEDURE	**(A)** The patient performs a bilateral straight leg raise to the height of 2 to 6 inches and is asked to hold the position for 30 seconds.
POSITIVE TEST	**(B)** The patient is unable to hold the position, cannot lift the leg, or experiences pain with the test.
IMPLICATIONS	Intrathecal or extrathecal pressure causing an intervertebral disc to place pressure on a lumbar nerve root.

Box 10–8 Kernig's test

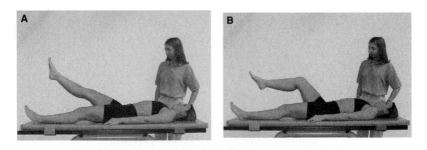

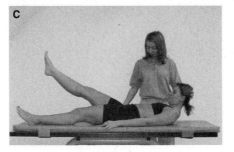

PATIENT POSITION	Supine
POSITION OF EXAMINER	At the side of the patient
EVALUATIVE PROCEDURE	The patient performs a unilateral active straight leg raise with the knee extended until pain occurs **(A)**. After pain occurs, the patient flexes the knee **(B)**.
POSITIVE TEST	Pain is experienced in the spine and possibly radiating into the lower extremity. This pain is relieved when the patient flexes the knee.
IMPLICATIONS	Nerve root impingement secondary to a bulging of the intervertebral disc or bony entrapment; irritation of the dural sheath; or irritation of the meninges.
MODIFICATION	In the absence of pain during the active straight leg raise, the examiner may further elongate the spinal cord and increase the tension on the dural sheath by passively flexing the patient's cervical spine **(Brudzinski's test)** and repeating the test **(C)**.

Box 10–9 Straight Leg Raise Test

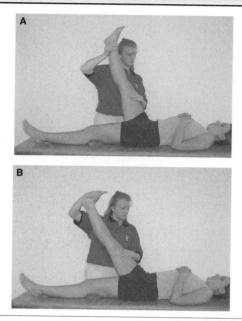

(A) The involved leg is flexed at the hip until symptoms are experienced. **(B)** The involved leg is extended approximately 10° (until symptoms subside) and the ankle is then passively dorsiflexed. A return of the symptoms indicates a stretching of the dural sheath.

PATIENT POSITION	Supine
POSITION OF EXAMINER	At the side to be tested; one hand grasps under the heel while the other is placed on the anterior knee to keep it in full extension during the examination.
EVALUATIVE PROCEDURE	While keeping the knee in extension, the examiner raises the leg by flexing the hip until discomfort is experienced or the full ROM is obtained.
POSITIVE TEST	The patient complains of pain before the end of the normal ROM (70°). The pain may be described as radiating distally along the tested leg, usually in the posterior thigh, radiating into the calf and perhaps the foot.
IMPLICATIONS	Sciatic nerve irritation Pain described before the hip reaches 70° of hip flexion may indicate discal involvement.
MODIFICATION	After pain is experienced, the leg is lowered to the point at which the pain stops. The examiner passively dorsiflexes the ankle and/or has the patient flex the cervical spine. Serving to stretch the dural sheath, this flexion recreates the symptoms. If the patient's prior pain was caused by tight hamstrings, this modification does not elicit pain.

ROM = range of motion.

Box 10–10 Well Straight Leg Raising Test

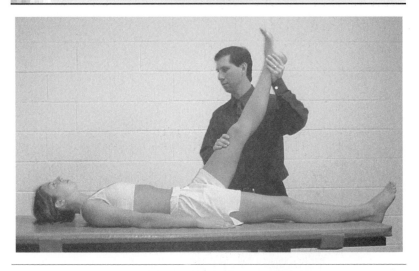

The well straight leg raise test differs from the straight leg raise test in that the unaffected leg is elevated.

PATIENT POSITION	Supine
POSITION OF EXAMINER	At the side to be tested (the extremity not suffering the symptoms); one hand grasps under the heel while the other is placed on the anterior thigh just superior to the knee to stabilize the leg in extension.
EVALUATIVE PROCEDURE	Keeping the knee in extension, the examiner raises the leg by flexing the hip until discomfort is reported.
POSITIVE TEST	Pain is experienced on the side opposite that being raised.
IMPLICATIONS	A large space-occupying lesion such as a herniated intervertebral disc

Box 10–11 Quadrant Test

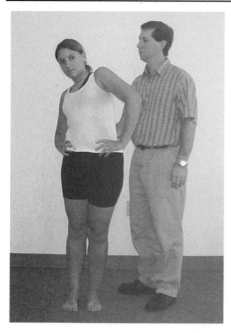

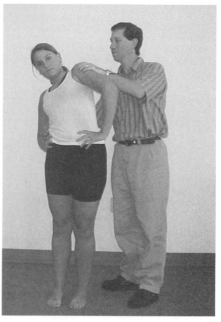

Box 10-11   Quadrant Test (Continued)

PATIENT POSITION	Standing with the feet shoulder width apart
POSITION OF EXAMINER	Standing behind the patient, grasping the patient's shoulders
EVALUATIVE PROCEDURE	The patient extends the spine as far as possible, then sidebends and rotates to the affected side. The examiner provides overpressure through the shoulders, supporting the patient as needed.
POSITIVE TEST	Reproduction of the patient's symptoms
IMPLICATIONS	Radicular pain indicates compression of the intervertebral foramina that impinges on the lumbar nerve roots. Local (nonradiating) pain indicates facet joint pathology. Symptoms isolated to the area of the PSIS; may also indicate SI joint dysfunction.

PSIS = posterior superior iliac spine; SI = sacroiliac.

Thorax and Lumbar

Box 10–12 Slump Test

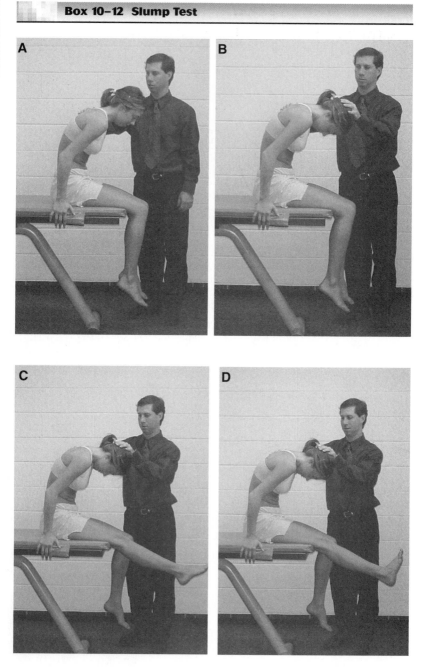

Box 10–12 **Slump Test** (Continued)	
PATIENT POSITION	Sitting over the edge of the table
POSITION OF EXAMINER	At the side of the patient
EVALUATIVE PROCEDURE	The following sequence is followed until symptoms are provoked: 1. The patient slumps forward along the thoracolumbar spine, rounding the shoulders while keeping the cervical spine in neutral **(A)**. 2. The patient flexes the cervical spine. The clinician then holds the patient in this position **(B)**. 3. The knee is actively extended **(C)**. 4. The ankle is actively dorsiflexed **(D)**. 5. Repeat steps 2 through 4 on the opposite side.
POSITIVE TEST	Sciatic pain or reproduction of other neurologic symptoms
IMPLICATIONS	Impingement of the dural lining, spinal cord, or nerve roots

Box 10–13 Hoover's Test

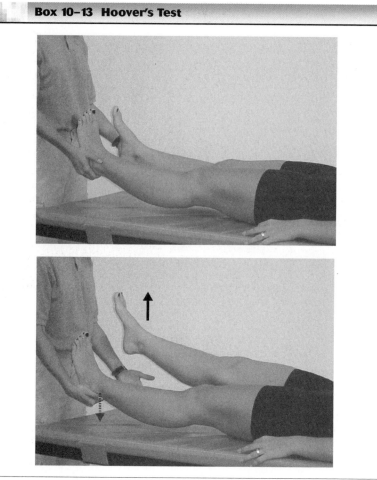

PATIENT POSITION	Supine
POSITION OF EXAMINER	At the feet of the patient with the evaluator's hands cupping the calcaneus of each leg
EVALUATIVE PROCEDURE	The patient attempts an active straight leg raise on the involved side
POSITIVE TEST	The patient does not attempt to lift the leg and the examiner does not sense pressure from the uninvolved leg pressing down on the hand as should instinctively happen.
IMPLICATION	The patient is not attempting to perform the test (i.e., malingering).

Box 10–14 Femoral Nerve Stretch Test

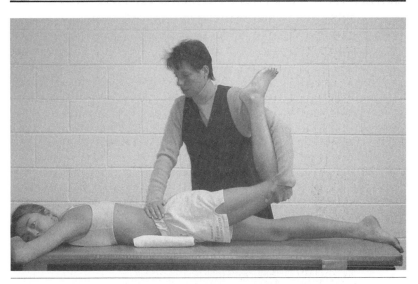

PATIENT POSITION	Prone with a pillow under the abdomen or sidelying
POSITION OF EXAMINER	At the side of the patient
EVALUATIVE PROCEDURE	The examiner passively extends the hip while keeping the patient's knee flexed to 90°.
POSITIVE TEST	Pain is elicited in the anterior and lateral thigh.
IMPLICATION	Nerve root impingement at the L2, L3, or L4 level
COMMENT	The examiner should attempt to fully flex the knee with the hip in the neutral position to determine any strain of the quadriceps muscle that may also cause pain.

Thorax and Lumbar

Box 10–15   Tension Sign   *Bowstring*

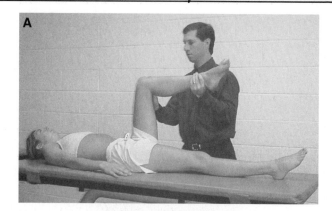

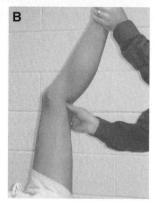

PATIENT POSITION	Supine
POSITION OF EXAMINER	At the patient's side that is to be tested; one hand grasps the heel while the other grasps the thigh.
EVALUATIVE PROCEDURE	The hip is flexed to 90°, with the knee flexed to 90°. The knee is then extended as far as possible with the examiner palpating the tibial portion of the sciatic nerve as it passes through the popliteal space **(A)**.
POSITIVE TEST	Exquisite tenderness with possible duplication of sciatic symptoms, as compared with the opposite side.
IMPLICATIONS	Sciatic nerve irritation
MODIFICATION	The **Bowstring test** is a variation of this technique **(B)**. The examiner extends the patient's knee until radiating symptoms are experienced. The knee is then flexed approximately 20° or until the symptoms are relieved. The examiner then pushes on the tibial portion of the sciatic nerve to reestablish the symptoms.

Box 10–16 Single Leg Stance Test

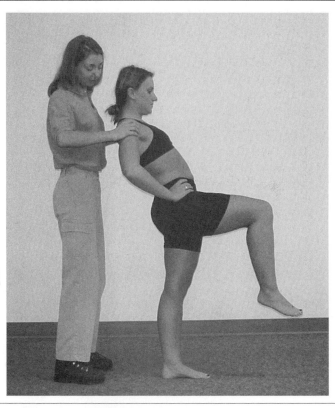

PATIENT POSITION	Standing with the body weight evenly distributed between the two feet
POSITION OF EXAMINER	Standing behind the patient, ready to provide support if the patient begins to fall
EVALUATIVE PROCEDURE	The patient lifts one leg, then places the trunk in hyperextension. The examiner may assist the patient during this motion. The procedure is then repeated for the opposite leg.
POSITIVE TEST	Pain is noted in the lumbar spine or SI area.
IMPLICATION	Shear forces are placed on the pars interarticularis by the iliopsoas pulling the vertebra anteriorly, resulting in pain.
COMMENTS	When the lesion to the pars interarticularis is unilateral, pain is evoked when the opposite leg is raised. Bilateral pars fractures result in pain when either leg is lifted. This test may exhibit pain specifically at the area of the PSIS secondary to SI joint irritation.

PSIS = posterior superior iliac spine; SI = sacroiliac.

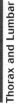

Box 10–17   Sacroiliac Joint Compression and Distraction Tests

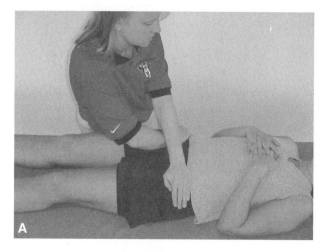

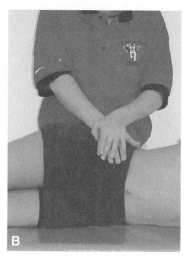

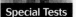

Box 10–17   Sacroiliac Joint Compression and Distraction Tests

(A) Sacroiliac joint compression test. Spreading the ASIS compresses the SI joint. **(B)** Sacroiliac joint distraction test. Compressing the ASIS distracts the SI joints. The distraction test should be performed on both sides.

PATIENT POSITION	Compression: Supine Distraction: Sidelying
POSITION OF EXAMINER	Compression: At the side of the patient with the hands placed over the opposite ASIS bilaterally Distraction: Behind the patient with both hands over the lateral aspect of the pelvis.
EVALUATIVE PROCEDURE	Compression: The examiner applies pressure to spread the ASIS, thus compressing the SI joints. Distraction: The examiner applies pressure down through the anterior portion of the ilium, spreading the SI joints.
POSITIVE TEST	Pain arising from the SI joint
IMPLICATIONS	Sacroiliac pathology

ASIS = anterior superior iliac spine; PSIS = posterior superior iliac spine; SI = sacroiliac.

Box 10–18   Fabere's Test

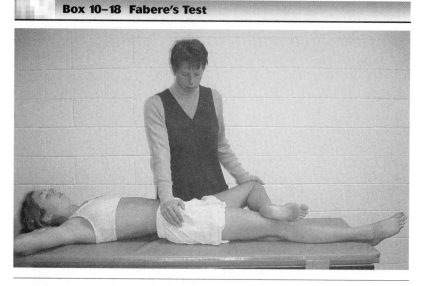

Fabere (flexion, abduction, external rotation, and extension) test for hip or sacroiliac pathology.

PATIENT POSITION	Supine, with the foot of the involved side crossed over the opposite thigh
POSITION OF EXAMINER	At the side of the patient to be tested with one hand on the opposite ASIS and the other on the medial aspect of the flexed knee
EVALUATIVE PROCEDURE	The extremity is allowed to rest into full external rotation followed by the examiner's applying overpressure at the knee and ASIS
POSITIVE TEST	Pain in the sacroiliac joint or hip
IMPLICATIONS	Pain in the inguinal area anterior to the hip may indicate hip pathology. Pain during the application of overpressure in the SI area may indicate SI joint pathology.

ASIS = anterior superior iliac spine; SI = sacroiliac.

Box 10–19 Gaenslen's Test

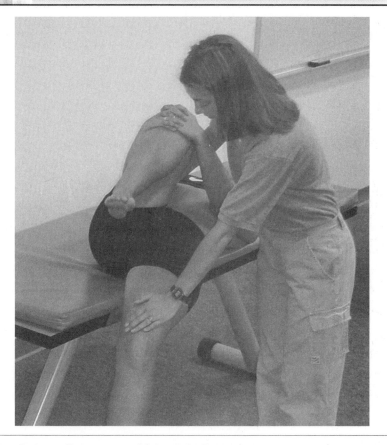

Gaenslen's test places a rotational force on·the SI joints.

PATIENT POSITION	Supine, lying close to the side of the table
POSITION OF EXAMINER	Standing at the side of the patient
EVALUATIVE PROCEDURE	The examiner slides the patient close to the edge of the table. The patient pulls the far knee up to the chest. The near leg is allowed to hang over the edge of the table.
POSITIVE TEST	While stabilizing the patient, the examiner applies pressure to the near leg, forcing it into hyperextension. The lumbar spine should not go into extension during this test. Pain in the SI region
IMPLICATIONS	SI joint dysfunction

SI = sacroiliac.

Box 10–20 Long Sit Test

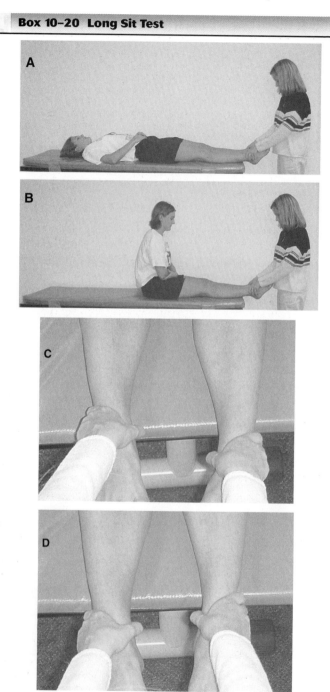

Box 10–20   Long Sit Test (Continued)

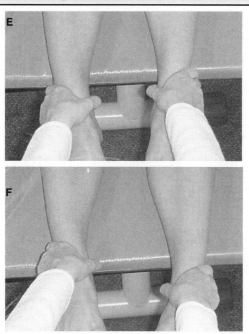

(A) Starting position. **(B)** Finishing position.
(C) Left leg is longer when supine and becomes shorter when assuming a sitting position.
(D) Signifying anterior rotation of the ilium.
(E) Left leg is shorter when supine and becomes longer when assuming a sitting position.
(F) Signifying posterior rotation of the ilium.

PATIENT POSITION	Supine with the heels off the table.
POSITION OF EXAMINER	Holding the feet with the thumbs placed over the medial malleoli.
EVALUATIVE PROCEDURE	The examiner provides slight traction on the legs while the patient arches and lifts the buttocks off the table. The patient then rests supine on the table. The patient then moves from a supine to a long sit position. The examiner must pay close attention to the position of the malleoli at all times throughout the test. This test is done actively if possible, without assistance provided by the upper extremities.
POSITIVE TEST	The movement of the medial malleoli is observed. If the involved leg (painful side) goes from a longer to a shorter position, there is an anterior rotation of the ilium on that side. If the involved side goes from a shorter to a longer position, posterior rotation of the ilium on the sacrum is indicated.
IMPLICATIONS	Rotated ilium as noted above.

Neurological Testing

Box 10–21 Lower Quarter Neurological Screen

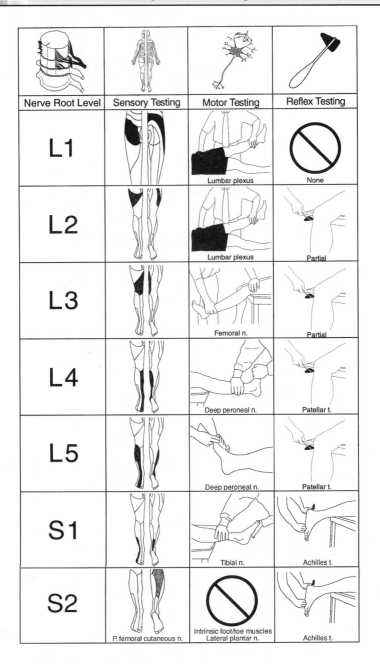

Nerve Root Level	Sensory Testing	Motor Testing	Reflex Testing
L1		Lumbar plexus	None
L2		Lumbar plexus	Partial
L3		Femoral n.	Partial
L4		Deep peroneal n.	Patellar t.
L5		Deep peroneal n.	Patellar t.
S1		Tibial n.	Achilles t.
S2	P. femoral cutaneous n.	Intrinsic foot/toe muscles Lateral plantar n.	Achilles t.

11

The Cervical Spine

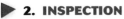

Cervical

Cervical Spine (Continued)

Lower motor neuron lesions
Upper quarter screen
Lower quarter screen

▶ **7. SPECIAL TESTS**

Brachial plexus pathology
Brachial plexus traction test

Cervical nerve root impingement
Shoulder abduction test
Cervical compression test
Spurling's test
Cervical distraction test

Vertebral artery test

AROM = active range of motion; PROM = passive range of motion; RROM = resisted range of motion.

History

Table 11–1 Possible Pathology Based on the Mechanism of Injury	
Mechanism	**Pathology**
Flexion	Compression of the anterior vertebral body and intervertebral disc Sprain of the supraspinous, interspinous, and posterior longitudinal ligaments and ligamentum flavum Sprain of the facet joints Strain of the posterior cervical musculature
Extension	Sprain of the anterior longitudinal ligament Compression of the posterior vertebral body and intervertebral disc Compression of the facet joints Fracture of the spinous processes

Lateral bending	On the side towards the bending:
	    Compression of the cervical nerve roots
	    Compression of the vertebral bodies and intervertebral disc
	    Compression of the facet joints
	On the side opposite the bending:
	    Stretching of the cervical nerve roots
	    Sprain of the lateral ligaments
	    Sprain of the facet joints
	    Strain of the cervical musculature

Rotation	Disc trauma Ligament sprain Facet sprain or dislocation Vertebral dislocation
Axial load	Compression fracture of the vertebral body Compression of the intervertebral disc

PALPATION

Palpation of the Anterior Cervical Spine Structures

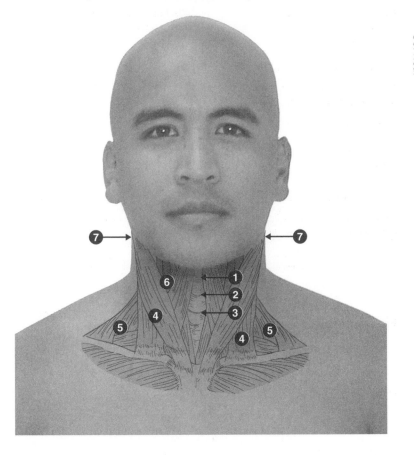

ANTERIOR CERVICAL SPINE

1 Hyoid bone
2 Thyroid cartilage
3 Cricoid cartilage
4 Sternocleidomastoid
5 Scalenes
6 Carotid artery
7 Lymph nodes

210   CHAPTER 11   The Cervical Spine

Palpation of the Posterior and Lateral Spine Structures

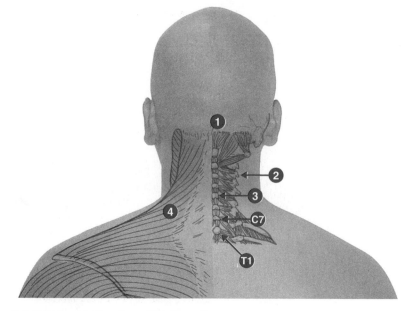

POSTERIOR AND LATERAL CERVICAL SPINE

1 Occiput and superior nuchal line
2 Transverse processes
3 Spinous processes
4 Trapezius

Table 11–2 Bony Landmarks for Palpation

Structure	Landmark
Cervical vertebral bodies	On the same level as the spinous processes
C1 transverse process	One finger's breadth inferior to the mastoid process
C3–C4 vertebrae	Posterior to the hyoid bone
C4–C5 vertebrae	Posterior to the thyroid cartilage
C6 vertebrae	Posterior to the cricoid cartilage; movement during flexion and extension of the cervical spine
C7 vertebra	Prominent posterior spinous process

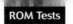

Range of Motion Testing

Measuring Cervical Spine Range of Motion

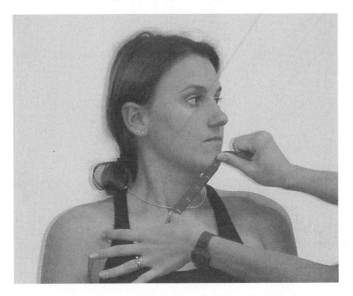

Figure 11–1 Measuring cervical range of motion with a tape measure. The distance from the jugular notch on the sternum to the point of the chin is measured and recorded for each motion. Cervical rotation is demonstrated in this photograph.

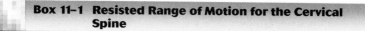

Cervical

Box 11–1 Resisted Range of Motion for the Cervical Spine

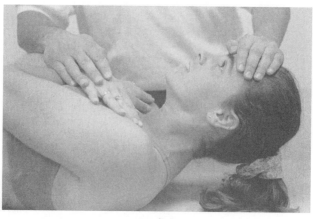

Flexion

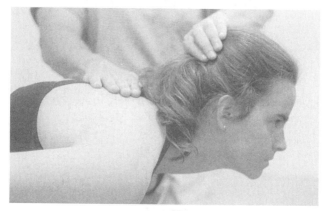

Extension

	Flexion	**Extension**
STARTING POSITION	Seated or supine with the cervical spine and head in the neutral position	Seated or prone with the cervical spine and head in the neutral position
STABILIZATION	Over the superior aspect of the sternum	Superior aspect of the thoracic spine (e.g., T2-T9)
RESISTANCE	To the forehead	To the skull over the occiput
MUSCLES TESTED	Sternocleidomastoid, anterior scalene	Trapezius (upper one third, levator scapulae, cervical paraspinal muscles (see Table 11–1)

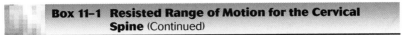

Box 11–1 Resisted Range of Motion for the Cervical Spine (Continued)

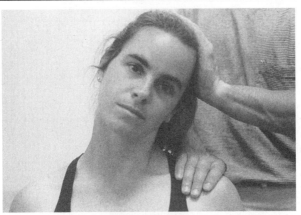

Lateral Flexion

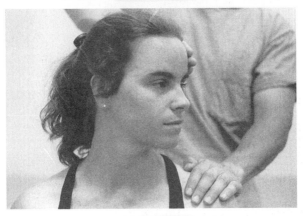

Rotation

	Lateral Flexion	**Rotation**
STARTING POSITION	Seated with the cervical spine and head in the neutral position	Seated with the cervical spine and head in the neutral position
STABILIZATION	Over the acromioclavicular joint on the side toward the motion	Over the anterior shoulder on the side toward the rotation
RESISTANCE	Over the temporal and parietal bones on the side toward the motion	Over the temporal bone on the side toward the motion
MUSCLES TESTED	Sternocleidomastoid, scalenes, paraspinal muscles on the side being tested	Sternocleidomastoid (opposite side), multifidus (opposite side), rotatores, upper trapezius (opposite side)

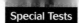
214   CHAPTER 11   The Cervical Spine

SPECIAL TESTS

Box 11–2 Brachial Plexus Traction Test

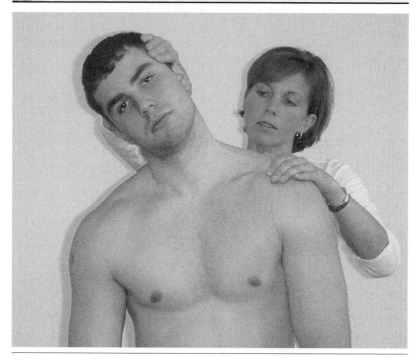

The examiner attempts to duplicate the mechanism of injury and replicate the patient's symptoms. Pain radiates down the patient's left shoulder when a traction injury exists and down the patient's right shoulder when a compression injury exists. This test should be duplicated in each direction and should not be performed until the possibility of cervical spine fracture or instability has been ruled out

PATIENT POSITION	Seated or standing
POSITION OF EXAMINER	Standing behind the patient
EVALUATIVE PROCEDURE	One hand placed on the side of the patient's head; the other hand placed over the acromioclavicular joint The cervical spine is laterally bent and the opposite shoulder depressed.
POSITIVE TEST	Pain radiating through the upper arm.
IMPLICATIONS	**Radiating pain on the side opposite the lateral bending:** Tension (stretching) of the brachial plexus **Radiating pain on the side toward the lateral bending:** Compression of the cervical nerve roots between two vertebrae
COMMENTS	This test should not be performed until the possibility of a cervical fracture or dislocation has been ruled out.

Box 11-3 Shoulder Abduction Test

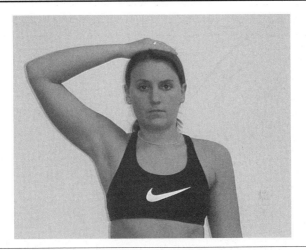

Because of its pain relieving qualities, the patient may assume this posture on his or her own.

PATIENT POSITION	Seated or standing
POSITION OF EXAMINER	Standing in front of the patient
EVALUATIVE PROCEDURE	The patient actively abducts the arm so that the hand is resting on top of the head.
POSITIVE TEST	Decrease in the patient's symptoms secondary to decreased tension on the involved nerve root
IMPLICATIONS	Herniated disc or nerve root compression

Spurlings

Box 11–4 Cervical Compression Test

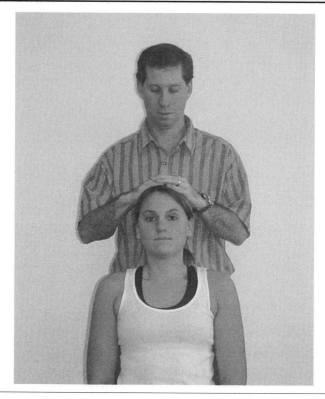

The cervical compression test attempts to duplicate the patient's symptoms by increasing pressure on the cervical nerve roots. This test should not be performed until cervical fracture, dislocation, or instability has been ruled out.

PATIENT POSITION	Sitting
POSITION OF EXAMINER	Standing behind the patient with hands interlocked over the top of the patient's head
EVALUATIVE PROCEDURE	The examiner presses down on the crown of the patient's head.
POSITIVE TEST	The patient experiences pain in the upper cervical spine, upper extremity, or both.
IMPLICATIONS	Compression of the facet joints and narrowing of the intervertebral foramen resulting in pain
COMMENTS	This test should not be performed until the possibility of a cervical fracture or instability has been ruled out.

Cervical

Box 11–5 Spurling's Test

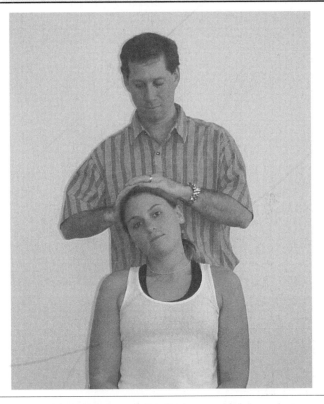

Similar to the cervical compression test, Spurling's test attempts to compress one of the cervical nerve roots. This test should not be performed until the possibility of a cervical fracture, dislocation, or instability has been ruled out.

PATIENT POSITION	Seated
POSITION OF EXAMINER	Standing behind the patient with the hands interlocked over the crown of the patient's head
EVALUATIVE PROCEDURE	The patient extends and laterally bends the cervical spine. A compressive force is then placed along the cervical spine.
POSITIVE TEST	Pain radiating down the patient's arm
IMPLICATIONS	Nerve root impingement by narrowing of the neural foramina
COMMENTS	This test should not be performed until the possibility of a cervical fracture or dislocation has been ruled out.

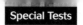
Cervical

Box 11–6 Cervical Distraction Test

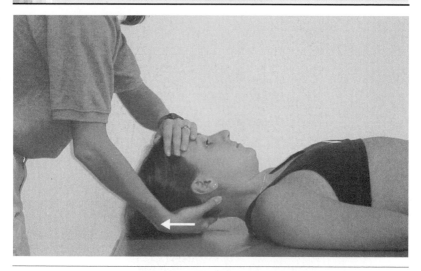

The cervical distraction test attempts to relieve the patient's symptoms by decreasing pressure on the cervical nerve roots. This test should not be performed until cervical fracture, dislocation, or instability has been ruled out.

PATIENT POSITION	Supine to relax the postural muscles of the cervical spine
POSITION OF EXAMINER	At the head of the patient with one hand under the occiput and the other on top of the forehead, stabilizing the head
EVALUATIVE PROCEDURE	The examiner applies traction on the patient's head, causing distraction of the cervical spine.
POSITIVE TEST	The patient's symptoms are relieved or reduced.
IMPLICATIONS	Compression of the cervical facet joints and/or stenosis of the neural foramina
COMMENTS	This test should not be performed until the possibility of a cervical fracture or dislocation has been ruled out.

Box 11–7 Vertebral Artery Test

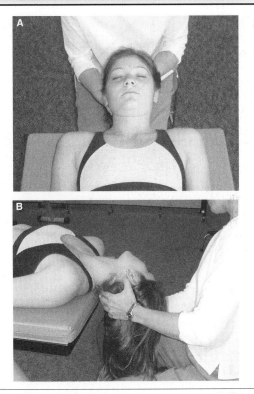

The vertebral artery test is performed to assure the competency of the vertebral artery prior to initiating treatment or rehabilitation techniques that may compromise a partially occluded artery. This test should not be performed until the presence of a cervical fracture, dislocation, or instability has been ruled out.

PATIENT POSITION	Supine
POSITION OF EXAMINER	Seated at the head of the patient with the hands placed under the occiput to stabilize the head
EVALUATIVE PROCEDURE	The examiner passively extends and laterally flexes the cervical spine **(A)**. The head is then rotated toward the laterally flexed side and held for 30 s **(B)**. During this procedure, the examiner must monitor the patient's pupillary activity.
POSITIVE TEST	Dizziness, confusion, nystagmus, unilateral pupil changes, nausea
IMPLICATIONS	Occlusion of the cervical vertebral arteries
COMMENTS	Patients with a positive test result should be referred to a physician before any other evaluative tests are performed or a rehabilitation plan is implemented and before being allowed to return to competition.

Neurological Testing

Cervical

Box 11–8 Upper Quarter Neurological Screen

Nerve Root Level	Sensory Testing	Motor Testing	Reflex Testing
C5	Axillary n.	Axillary n.	Biceps brachii
C6	Musculocutaneous n.	Musculocutaneous n. (C5 & C6)	Brachioradialis
C7	Radial n.	Radial n.	Triceps brachii
C8	Ulnar n. (mixed)	Median & palm. interosseous n.	None
T1	Med. brachial cutaneous n.	None	None

Box 11–9 Babinski's Test for Upper Motor Neuron Lesions

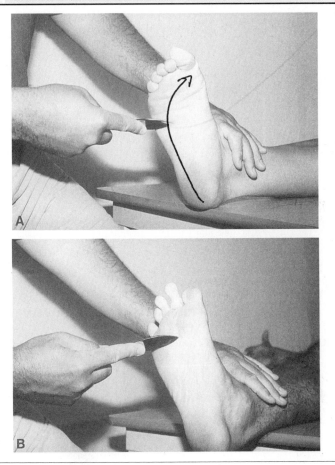

The Babinski test is most commonly performed during the evaluation of an acute head or cervical spine injury to determine the presence of an upper motor neuron lesion.

PATIENT POSITION	Supine.
POSITION OF EXAMINER	At the foot of the patient; a blunt device, such as the handle of a reflex hammer or the handle of a pair of scissors, is needed.
EVALUATIVE PROCEDURE	The examiner runs the device up the plantar aspect of the foot, making an arc from the calcaneus medially to the ball of the great toe (**A**). *curling = tickling*
POSITIVE TEST	The great toe extends and the other toes splay (**B**). *= upper motor neuron lesion*
IMPLICATIONS	Upper motor neuron lesion, especially in the pyramidal tract, caused by brain or spinal cord trauma or pathology
COMMENTS	The Babinski reflex occurs normally in newborns and should spontaneously disappear shortly after birth.

upper motor neuron is below brain stem

Cervical

Box 11–10 Oppenheim's Test for Upper Motor Neuron Lesions

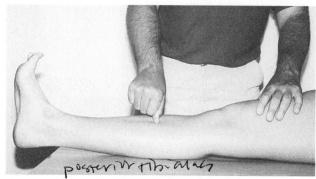

posterior Tibialis

The Oppenheim test is most commonly performed during the evaluation of a patient with acute head or cervical spine injury to determine the presence of an upper motor neuron lesion.

PATIENT POSITION	Supine
POSITION OF EXAMINER	At the patient's side
EVALUATIVE PROCEDURE	The examiner's fingernail is run along the crest of the anteromedial tibia.
POSITIVE TEST	The great toe extends and the other toes splay or the patient reports hypersensitivity to the test.
IMPLICATIONS	Upper motor neuron lesion caused by brain or spinal cord trauma or pathology

BILATERAL

12

The Thorax and Abdomen

EVALUATION MAP:
Thorax and Abdomen

 1. HISTORY

Location of pain

Onset of symptoms

Mechanism of injury

Symptoms

History

General medical health

 2. INSPECTION

Guarding pattern

Breathing pattern

Discoloration of skin

Vomiting

Hematuria

Auscultation

3. PALPATION

Sternum
Xiphoid process
Sternal body

Costal cartilage

Ribs

Spleen

Kidneys

Appendix
McBurney's point

4. VITAL SIGNS

Heart rate

Respiratory rate

Blood pressure

5. NEUROLOGIC TESTS

Referred pain patterns

6. SPECIAL TESTS

Kidney function
Urinalysis

Abdominal injury
Abdominal percussion

Rib fractures
Compression test

History

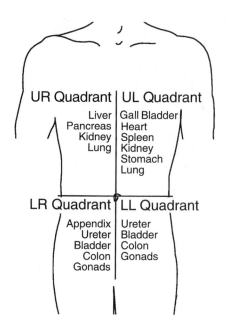

Figure 12–1 Abdominal quadrant reference system. The sagittal quadrants are relative to the athlete. Therefore, the right kidney is on the athlete's right-hand side.

| | Quadrant Segment (Relative to the Patient) | |
	Right	Left
Upper	**Liver:** Pain is associated with **cholecystitis** or liver laceration. **Gallbladder:** Pain without the history of trauma indicates gallbladder disease.	**Spleen:** Rigidity under the last several ribs indicates trauma to the spleen.
Lower	**Appendix:** Rebound tenderness indicates appendicitis. **Colon:** Colitis or diverticulitis may cause pain. **Pelvic inflammation** results in diffuse tenderness.	**Colon:** Colitis or diverticulitis may cause pain. **Pelvic inflammation** results in diffuse tenderness.

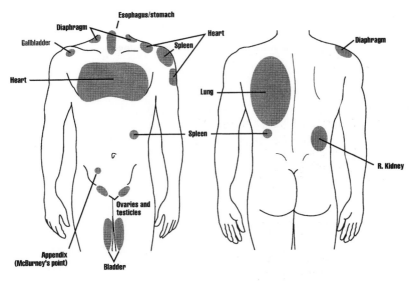

Figure 12–2 Referred pain patterns from the viscera. Pain from the internal organs tends to radiate along the corresponding somatic sensory fibers.

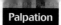
PALPATION

Palpation of the Thorax and Abdomen

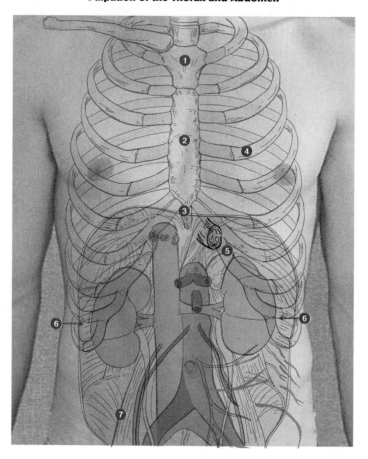

STERNUM

1 Manubrium

2 Sternal body

3 Xiphoid process

4 Costal cartilage and ribs

5 Spleen

6 Kidneys

7 McBurney's point

Location of McBurney's Point

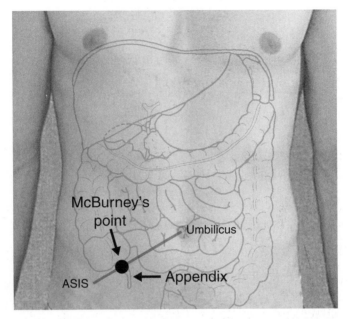

Figure 12–3 McBurney's point, located approximately one-third of the way between the ASIS and the umbilicus. This point becomes tender in the presence of appendicitis.

Box 12–1 "Clean Catch" Dipstick Urinalysis

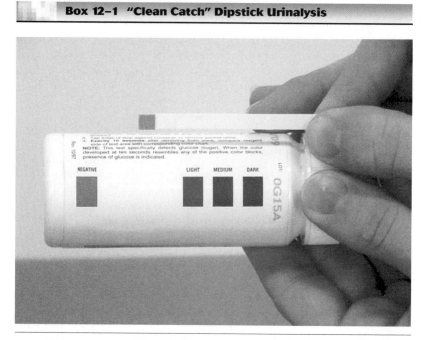

EVALUATIVE PROCEDURE

The external urethra and surrounding area is cleansed using soap and water and then rinsed.

To clear the urethra, the initial flow of urine is into a toilet bowl or "dirty" collection container.

One to 2 oz of urine are then collected in a clean specimen cup.

The dipstick is then immersed into the specimen cup.

The manufacturer's recommendations for immersion time and interpretation times are followed.

Box 12-1   "Clean Catch" Dipstick Urinalysis

TEST RESULTS	The colors produced on the dipstick are matched to the values provided by the manufacturer.		
IMPLICATIONS	**Element**	**Normal**	**Interpretation**
	Specific gravity	1.006 to 1.030	**Low reading:** Diabetes mellitus, excessive hydration, renal failure
			High reading: Dehydration; heart or renal failure
	pH	4.6 to 8.0	**Low reading:** Chronic obstructive pulmonary disease, diabetic ketoacidosis
			High reading: Renal failure, urinary tract infection
	Glucose, gld	<0.5	Diabetes, stress
	Ketones	0	Anorexia, poor nutrition, alcoholism, diabetes mellitus
	Protein	0	Congestive heart failure, polycystic kidney disease
	Hemoglobin	0	Urinary tract infection, kidney disease or trauma
	RBC	0	Kidney disease or trauma, kidney stones, bladder infection, urinary tract infection
COMMENTS	The above interpretations are partial lists. High or low readings should be interpreted by a physician. Factors such as diet and the level of exercise can alter the urinalysis readings.		

RBC = red blood cell.

Thorax and Abdomen

Box 12–2 Abdominal Percussion

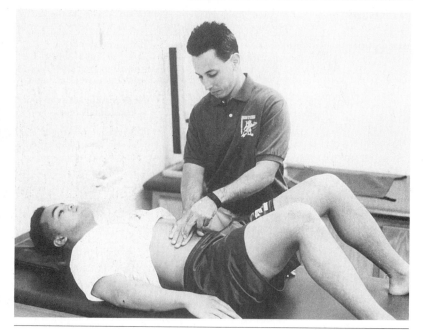

PATIENT POSITION	Hook lying
POSITION OF EXAMINER	Standing to the patient's side The examiner lightly places one hand palm down over the area to be assessed The index and middle fingers of the opposite hand tap the DIP joints of the hand placed over the athlete's abdomen
EVALUATIVE PROCEDURE	The fingertips of the top hand quickly strike the middle phalanges of the bottom hand in a tapping motion. The sound of the echo within the abdomen is noted. Areas over solid organs have a dull thump associated with them. Hollow organs make a crisper, more **resonant** sound.
POSITIVE TEST	A hard, solid sounding echo over areas that should normally sound hollow.
IMPLICATIONS	Internal bleeding filling the abdominal cavity.

DIP = distal interphalangeal.

Box 12-3 Determination of Heart Rate Using the Carotid Pulse

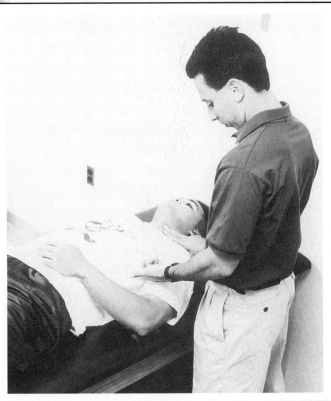

PATIENT POSITION	Seated or lying down
POSITION OF EXAMINER	Using the index and middle fingers to locate the thyroid cartilage, move the fingers laterally in either direction to find the common carotid artery between the thyroid cartilage and the sternocleidomastoid muscle.
EVALUATIVE PROCEDURE	Count the number of pulses in a 15-s interval and multiply that number by 4 to determine the number of beats per minute. The examiner also attempts to determine the quality of the pulse: strong (bounding) or weak.
POSITIVE TEST	Not applicable
IMPLICATIONS	The quality and quantity of the heart rate established. **Normal (general population):** 60 to 100 bpm **Well-trained athletes:** 40 to 60 bpm **Tachycardia:** Greater than 100 bpm **Bradycardia:** Less than 60 bpm
COMMENTS	The baseline heart rate should be recorded and rechecked at regular intervals.

bpm = beats per minute.

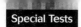

Thorax and Abdomen

Box 12-4 Blood Pressure Assessment

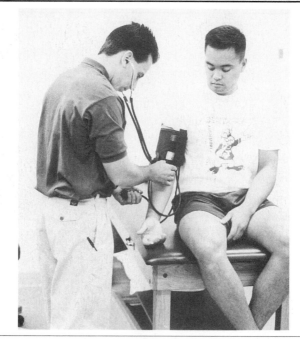

PATIENT POSITION	Seated or lying supine
POSITION OF EXAMINER	In front of or beside the patient in a position to read the gauge on the BP cuff.
EVALUATIVE PROCEDURE	The cuff is secured over the upper arm. Many cuffs have an arrow that must be aligned with the brachial artery. The stethoscope is placed over the brachial artery. The cuff is inflated to 180 to 200 mm Hg. The air is slowly released from the cuff. While reading the gauge, note the point at which the first pulse sound, the systolic pressure, is heard. Continuing to slowly release the air from the cuff, note the value at which the last pulse, the diastolic value, is heard.
POSITIVE TEST	A systolic value below 100 mm Hg or above 140 mm Hg A diastolic value below 65 mm Hg or above 90 mm Hg
IMPLICATIONS	Low BP may indicate shock or internal hemorrhage High BP indicates hypertension
COMMENTS	The athlete's baseline BP should be obtained annually during the preparticipation physical examination and should be compared with the current readings. Larger patients may require the use of a larger BP cuff. A cuff that is too small erroneously increases the BP.

BP = blood pressure.

Box 12–5 Compression Test for Rib Fractures

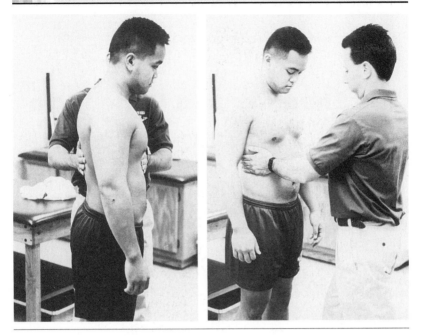

PATIENT POSITION	Seated or standing
POSITION OF EXAMINER	Standing in front of the patient with the hands on opposite sides of the rib cage.
EVALUATIVE PROCEDURE	The examiner compresses the rib cage in an anterior-posterior direction and quickly releases the pressure. The rib cage is then compressed from the patient's side and the pressure is quickly released.
POSITIVE TEST	Pain in the rib cage
IMPLICATIONS	Damage to the rib cage, including the possibility of a fracture, contusion, or costochondral separation.

13

The Shoulder and Upper Arm

EVALUATION MAP: Shoulder

 1. HISTORY

Location of the pain
Onset
Activity
Injury mechanism
Symptoms
Prior injury

 2. INSPECTION

General
The position of the head
The position of the arm

Anterior Structures
Level of the shoulders
Contour of the clavicles
Symmetry of the deltoid muscle
   groups
Anterior humerus
Biceps brachii

Lateral Structures
Deltoid muscle group
Acromion process
   Step deformity
Position of the humerus

Posterior Structures
Alignment of the spinal vertebrae
Position of the scapula
Muscle tone
Position of the humerus

 3. PALPATION

Anterior Structures
Jugular notch
SC ligament
Clavicular shaft
Acromion process
   Piano key sign
Coracoid process
Pectoralis major
Pectoralis minor
Deltoid muscle group

Humerus
Humeral head
Greater/lesser tuberosities
Bicipital groove
Humeral shaft
Coracobrachialis
Biceps brachii
   Long head tendon
   Short head tendon

Scapula
Spine of the scapula
Superior angle
Inferior angle
Rotator cuff
Teres major
Rhomboids
Levator scapulae
Trapezius
Latissimus dorsi
Triceps brachii

▶ 4. RANGE OF MOTION TESTS

Active Range of Motion
Apley's scratch test
Flexion
Extension
    Gerber lift-off test
Abduction
Adduction
Internal rotation
External rotation
Horizontal adduction
Horizontal abduction

Passive Range of Motion
Flexion
Extension
Abduction
Adduction
Internal rotation
External rotation
Horizontal adduction
Horizontal abduction

Resisted Range of Motion
Flexion
Extension
Abduction
Adduction
Internal rotation
External rotation
Horizontal adduction
Horizontal abduction

Scapular Movements
Elevation
Depression
Retraction
Protraction
Rotation

▶ 5. LIGAMENTOUS TESTS

SC glide
AC glide
GH joint
    Apprehension test
    GH glide

▶ 6. NEUROLOGICAL TESTS

Brachial plexus
Cervical nerve root

Thoracic outlet syndrome
Adson's test
Allen's test
Military brace position

▶ 7. SPECIAL TESTS

Acromioclavicular joint sprain
AC traction test
AC compression test

Glenohumeral pathology
Relocation test
Posterior apprehension test
Posterior apprehension test in the
    plane of the scapula
Sulcus sign
Active compression test

Rotator cuff pathology
Drop arm test
Neer impingement test
Hawkins shoulder impingement test
Empty can test

Biceps tendon pathology
Yergason's test
Speed's test
Ludington's test

Shoulder and Arm

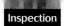
236   C H A P T E R   1 3   The Shoulder and Upper Arm

Inspection

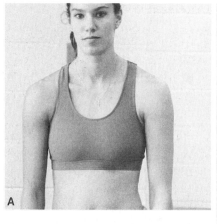
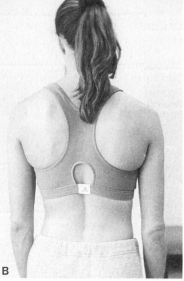

Figure 13–1 (**A**) Anterior and (**B**) posterior view of the shoulders. Note that the shoulder of the dominant right arm hangs lower than the shoulder of the nondominant arm.

PALPATION

Palpation of Anterior Shoulder

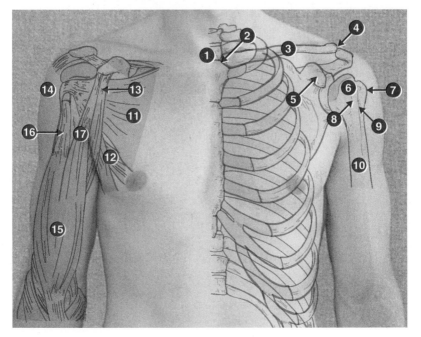

ANTERIOR SHOULDER

1 Jugular notch	10 Humeral shaft
2 Sternoclavicular joint	11 Pectoralis major
3 Clavicular shaft	12 Pectoralis minor
4 Acromion process and AC joint	13 Coracobrachialis
5 Coracoid process	14 Deltoid muscle group
6 Humeral head	15 Biceps brachii muscle
7 Greater tuberosity	16 Long head of the biceps tendon
8 Lesser tuberosity	17 Short head of the biceps tendon
9 Bicipital groove	

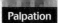

Palpation of Posterior Shoulder

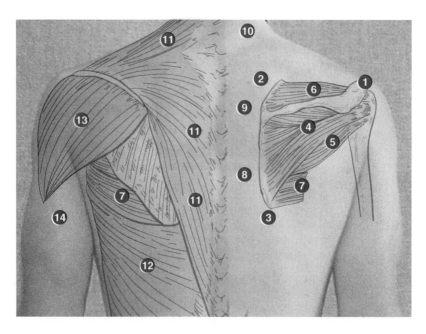

POSTERIOR SHOULDER

  1 Spine of the scapula

  2 Superior angle of the scapula

  3 Inferior angle of the scapula

ROTATOR CUFF MUSCLES (4–6)

      4 Infraspinatus

      5 Teres minor

      6 Supraspinatus

  7 Teres major

  8 Rhomboid major

  9 Rhomboid minor

10 Levator scapula

11 Trapezius

12 Latissimus dorsi

13 Posterior deltoid

14 Triceps brachii

Shoulder and Arm

Range of Motion Testing

Box 13–1   Shoulder Goniometry

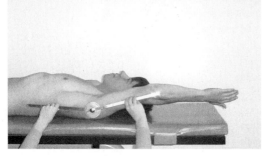

Flexion

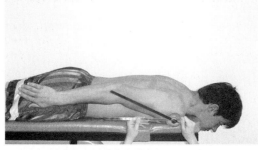

Extension

	Flexion	**Extension**
PATIENT POSITION	Supine	Prone
GONIOMETER PLACEMENT		
FULCRUM	Aligned lateral to the acromion process	Aligned lateral to the acromion process
STATIONARY ARM	Aligned parallel to the table top	Aligned parallel to the table top
MOVEMENT ARM	Centered over the midline of the lateral humerus	Centered over the midline of the lateral humerus

Box 13–1   Shoulder Goniometry (Continued)

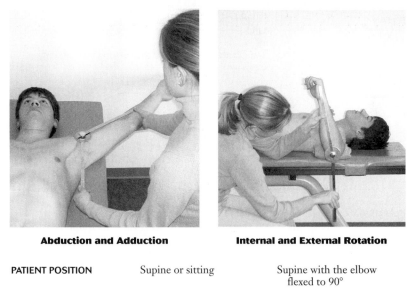

Abduction and Adduction   **Internal and External Rotation**

	Abduction and Adduction	**Internal and External Rotation**
PATIENT POSITION	Supine or sitting	Supine with the elbow flexed to 90°
GONIOMETER PLACEMENT		
FULCRUM	Anterior to the acromion process	Centered lateral to the olecranon process
STATIONARY ARM	Parallel to the long axis of the torso	Perpendicular to the floor or parallel to the tabletop
MOVEMENT ARM	Centered over the midline of the anterior humerus	Centered over the long axis of the ulna

Shoulder and Arm

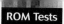

Table 13–1 Shoulder-Capsular Patterns and End-Feels

Capsular Pattern (glenohumeral joint): External rotation, abduction, internal rotation

Elevation	Firm–	Stretch of the glenohumeral 1. (middle and inferior bands); inferior joint capsule; latissimus dorsi; pectoralis major
	Hard–	Bony contact between the greater tuberosity and the acromion process (often pathological)
Extension	Firm–	Stretch of the coracohumeral 1. (anterior band); anterior joint capsule
Flexion	Firm–	Stretch of the coracohumeral 1. (posterior band); posterior capsule; teres minor; teres major; infraspinatus
Abduction	Firm–	Stretch of the glenohumeral 1. (middle and inferior bands); inferior joint capsule; latissimus dorsi; pectoralis major
	Hard–	Bony contact between the greater tuberosity and the acromion process (often pathological)
Horizontal abduction	Firm–	Stretch of the anterior capsule; glenohumeral 1.; coracohumeral 1; pectoralis major; coracobrachialis
Horizontal adduction	Firm–	Stretch of the posterior joint capsule; teres minor; teres major; infraspinatus
	Soft–	Contact between the pectoralis major and anterior deltoid
Internal rotation	Firm–	Stretch of the posterior joint capsule; infraspinatus; teres minor
External rotation	Firm–	Stretch of the glenohumeral 1.; coracohumeral 1.; anterior capsule; subscapularis; pectoralis major; latissimus dorsi; teres major

Shoulder and Arm

Shoulder Range of Motion:
Flexion and Extension

Shoulder Range of Motion:
Abduction and Adduction

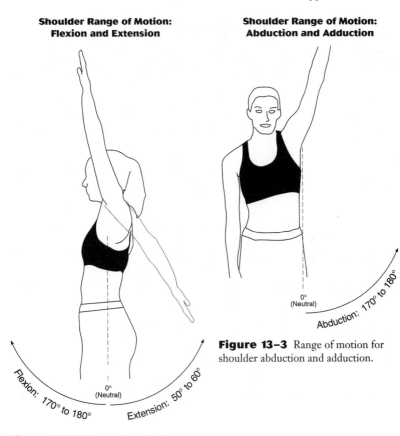

Abduction: 170° to 180°

0°
(Neutral)

Figure 13–3 Range of motion for
shoulder abduction and adduction.

Flexion: 170° to 180°

0°
(Neutral)

Extension: 50° to 60°

Figure 13–2 Range of motion for
shoulder flexion and extension.

Shoulder Range of Motion:
Internal and External Rotation

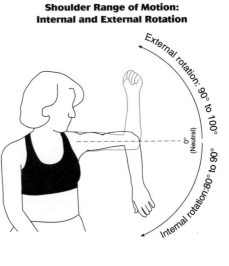

External rotation: 90° to 100°

0°
(Neutral)

Internal rotation:80° to 90°

Figure 13–4 Range of motion
for shoulder internal rotation and
external rotation.

Box 13–2 Apley's Scratch Tests

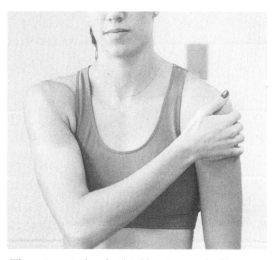

The patient touches the shoulder opposite the front
Motions produced: GH adduction, horizontal adduction,
  and internal rotation; scapular protraction

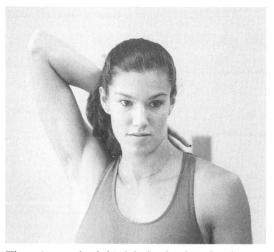

The patient reaches behind the head and touches the
  opposite shoulder from behind
Motions produced: GH abduction and external rotation;
  scapular protracton, elevation, and upward rotation

Shoulder and Arm

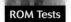

Box 13-2 Apley's Scratch Tests (Continued)

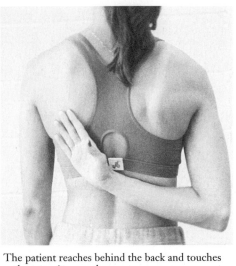

The patient reaches behind the back and touches
the opposite scapula
Motions produced: GH adduction and internal
rotation; scapular retraction and downward
rotation

GH = glenohumeral

Shoulder and Arm

Box 13–3   Resisted Range of Motion for the Shoulder

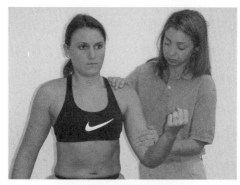

Flexion and Extension

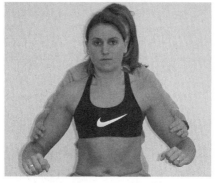

Abduction and Adduction

	Flexion and Extension	Abduction and Adduction
STARTING POSITION	Seated The humerus in the neutral position	Seated The humerus abducted to approximately 30°
STABILIZATION	Superior aspect of the shoulder	The torso, possibly although the patient's body weight may be sufficient
RESISTANCE	Distal humerus, just proximal to the elbow on the side toward the motion being tested	Distal humerus, just proximal to the elbow on the side toward the motion being tested
MUSCLES TESTED	**Flexion:** anterior deltoid, pectoralis major (clavicular portion), coracobrachialis, middle deltoid, biceps brachii	**Abduction:** deltoid muscle group, supraspinatus, biceps brachii
	Extension: posterior deltoid, latissimus dorsi, teres major, triceps brachii (long head)	**Adduction:** pectoralis major, coracobrachialis, latissimus dorsi, teres major, triceps brachii

Box 13-3 Resisted Range of Motion for the Shoulder (Continued)

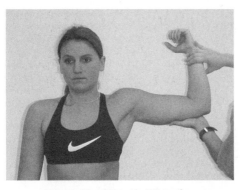

Internal and External Rotation

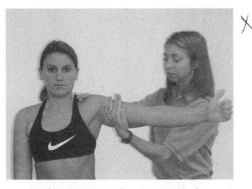

Horizontal Abduction and Adduction

Shoulder and Arm

	Internal and External Rotation	**Horizontal Abduction and Adduction**
STARTING POSITION	Seated The humerus in neutral position or abducted to 90° The elbow flexed to 90°	Seated or supine The elbow extended
STABILIZATION	The distal humerus is stabilized just proximal to the elbow.	Superior aspect of the shoulder (if needed)
RESISTANCE	Distal forearm on the side toward the motion being tested	Mid-humerus on the side toward the motion being tested
MUSCLES TESTED	**Internal rotation:** anterior deltoid, latissimus dorsi, pectoralis major, subscapularis, teres major **External rotation:** posterior deltoid, infraspinatus, supraspinatus, teres minor	**Horizontal abduction:** posterior deltoid, infraspinatus, teres minor **Horizontal adduction:** anterior deltoid, pectoralis major

Box 13–4 Gerber's Lift-off Test for Subscapularis Weakness

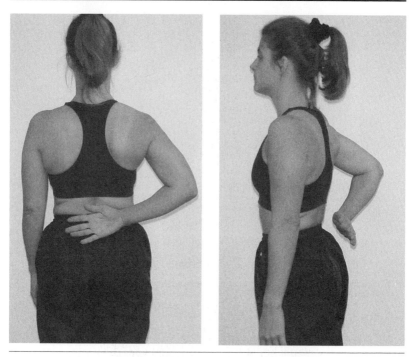

PATIENT POSITION	Standing with the humerus internally rotated
	The dorsal surface of the hand placed against the mid-lumbar spine
POSITION OF EXAMINER	Standing behind the patient
EVALUATIVE PROCEDURE	The patient attempts to actively lift the hand off the spine while the humerus stays in extension.
POSITIVE TEST	The inability to lift the hand off the spine
IMPLICATIONS	Positive test findings are associated with tears and weakness of the subscapularis muscle.
MODIFICATION	Resistance can be applied to the patient's palm.

Shoulder and Arm

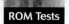

Box 13-5 Manual Muscle Testing of the Scapular Muscles

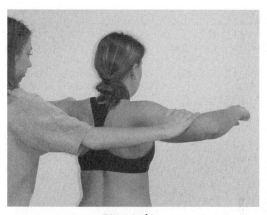

Rhomboids

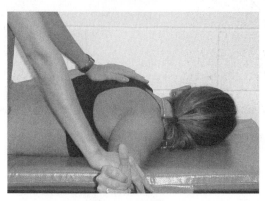

Middle Trapezius

Shoulder and Arm

	Rhomboids	**Middle Trapezius**
STARTING POSITION	While in the seated position, the elbow is flexed; the humerus is adducted and slightly extended.	In the prone position, the elbow is extended and the humerus is abducted to 90° and externally rotated so that the thumb points upward.
STABILIZATION	Not applicable	Not applicable
RESISTANCE	The examiner attempts to horizontally abduct the humerus while noting for scapular protraction indicating weakness.	A downward pressure is applied to the distal humerus.

Ligamentous Tests

Box 13–6 Glenohumeral Glide Tests

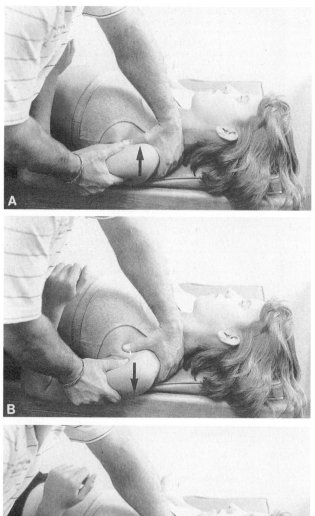

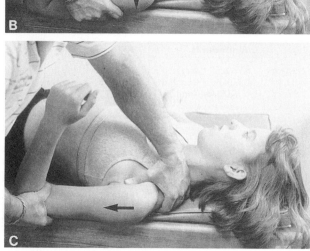

Box 13-6 Glenohumeral Glide Tests (Continued)	
PATIENT POSITION	Lying supine with the GH joint over the edge of the table
POSITION OF EXAMINER	Standing lateral to the side being tested with one hand stabilizing the shoulder complex by grasping the scapula and the other grasping the humerus just below the surgical neck.
EVALUATIVE PROCEDURE	The examiner applies a gentle, yet firm force that moves the humeral head anteriorly relative to the glenoid fossa while applying a slight distraction to the joint to separate the humeral head from the fossa. This procedure is then repeated in the posterior and inferior direction.
POSITIVE TEST	Pain or increased motion compared with the same direction on the opposite shoulder.
IMPLICATIONS	Laxity of the static stabilizers of the GH joint: **(A) Anterior:** coracohumeral ligament, superior and middle GH ligaments, anterior joint capsule, labral tear **(B) Posterior:** posterior joint capsule, labral tear. **(C) Inferior-anterior:** inferior joint capsule, superior GH ligament, coracohumeral ligament
MODIFICATION	In the case of large patients, a second examiner can be used to assist in stabilizing the scapula.

GH = glenohumeral.

Shoulder and Arm

SPECIAL TESTS

Box 13–7 Drop Arm Test for Rotator Cuff Tears

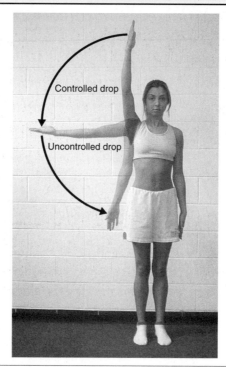

Controlled drop

Uncontrolled drop

PATIENT POSITION	Standing or sitting The humerus fully abducted and externally rotated and the forearm supinated
POSITION OF EXAMINER	Standing lateral to, or behind, the involved extremity
EVALUATIVE PROCEDURE	The patient slowly lowers the arm to the side
POSITIVE TEST	The arm falls uncontrollably from a position of approximately 90° abduction to the side
IMPLICATIONS	The inability to lower the arm in a controlled manner is indicative of lesions to the rotator cuff, especially the supraspinatus.
MODIFICATION	If the patient is able to lower the arm in a controlled manner through the ROM, a derivative of the drop arm test may be implemented: • The patient holds the humerus in 90° abduction. • The examiner applies gentle pressure on the distal forearm. • A positive test result causes the arm to fall against the side of the body, indicating lesions to the rotator cuff

ROM = range of motion.

Box 13–8   Apprehension Test for Anterior Glenohumeral Laxity

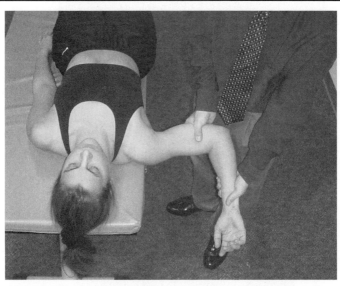

PATIENT POSITION	Supine, standing, or sitting The GH joint abducted to 90° and the elbow flexed to 90°
POSITION OF EXAMINER	Positioned in front of or beside the patient on the involved side The examiner supporting the humerus at midshaft while the forearm is grasped proximal to the wrist
EVALUATIVE PROCEDURE	While supporting the humerus at 90° abduction, the examiner passively externally rotates the GH joint by slowly applying pressure to the anterior forearm.
POSITIVE TEST	The patient displays apprehension that the shoulder may dislocate and resists further movement. Pain is centered in the anterior capsule of the GH joint.
IMPLICATIONS	The anterior capsule, inferior GH ligament, or glenoid labrum have been compromised, allowing the humeral head to dislocate or subluxate anteriorly on the glenoid fossa.
CAUTION	Pressure should be applied gradually and the test terminated at the first sign of apprehension. Do not perform this test when there is obvious dislocation or subluxation of the GH joint

GH = glenohumeral.

Shoulder and Arm

Box 13–9 Acromioclavicular Traction Test

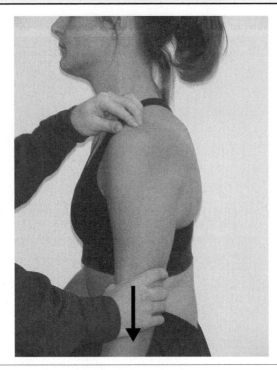

The principle behind the AC traction test is similar to a stress radiograph used to diagnose AC instability.

PATIENT POSITION	Sitting or standing The arm hanging naturally from the side
POSITION OF EXAMINER	Standing lateral to the involved side The clinician grasps the patient's humerus proximal to the elbow. The opposite hand gently palpates the AC joint.
EVALUATIVE PROCEDURE	The examiner applies a downward traction on the humerus.
POSITIVE TEST	The humerus and scapula move inferior to the clavicle, causing a step deformity, pain, or both.
IMPLICATIONS	Sprain of the AC or coracoclavicular ligaments
COMMENT	Patients displaying positive AC traction test results should be referred to a physician for follow-up radiographic stress testing and to rule out a clavicular fracture.

AC = acromioclavicular.

Box 13-10 Acromioclavicular Compression Test

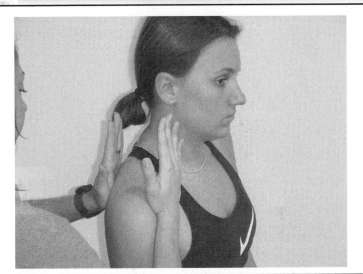

PATIENT POSITION	Sitting or standing with the arm hanging naturally at the side
POSITION OF EXAMINER	Standing on the involved side with the hands cupped over the anterior and posterior joint structures
EVALUATIVE PROCEDURE	The examiner squeezes the hands together, compressing the AC joint.
POSITIVE TEST	Pain at the AC joint or excursion of the clavicle over the acromion process
IMPLICATIONS	Damage to the AC ligament and possibly the coracoclavicular ligament.

AC = acromioclavicular.

Box 13–11 Relocation Test for Anterior Glenohumeral Laxity

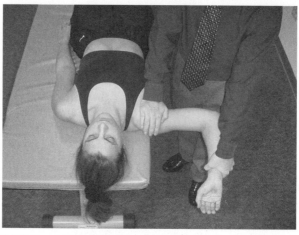

PATIENT POSITION	Supine The GH joint abducted to 90° The elbow flexed to 90°
POSITION OF EXAMINER	Standing beside the patient, inferior to the humerus on the involved side The forearm grasped proximal to the wrist to provide leverage during external rotation of the humerus The opposite hand held over the humeral head
EVALUATIVE PROCEDURE	The examiner externally rotates the humerus until pain, discomfort, or apprehension of a dislocation is experienced by the patient or the normal ROM is met. Posterior pressure is then applied to relocate the subluxated joint.
POSITIVE TEST	Decreased pain or increased ROM (or both) compared with the anterior apprehension test
IMPLICATIONS	Anterior pain may be the result of increased laxity in the anterior ligamentous and capsular structures. Posterior pain may be from the impingement of the posterior capsule or labrum. A positive test result supports the conclusion of increased laxity in the anterior capsule owing to capsular damage or labrum tears. The manual pressure applied by the examiner increases the stability of the anterior portion of the GH capsule, allowing more external rotation to occur.
COMMENT	The relocation test is usually performed after the anterior apprehension test.

GH = glenohumeral; ROM = range of motion.

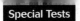
Box 13-12 Posterior Apprehension Test for Glenohumeral Laxity

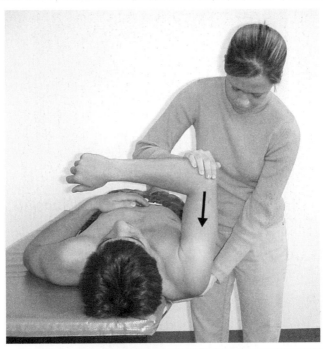

PATIENT POSITION	Sitting or supine The shoulder flexed to 90° and the elbow flexed to 90° The GH joint being tested off to the side of the table
POSITION OF EXAMINER	Standing on the involved side One hand grasping the forearm The opposite hand stabilizing the posterior scapula
EVALUATIVE PROCEDURE	The examiner applies a longitudinal force to the humeral shaft, encouraging the humeral head to move posteriorly on the glenoid fossa. The examiner may choose to alter the amount of flexion and rotation of the humerus.
POSITIVE TEST	The patient displays apprehension and produces muscle guarding to prevent the shoulder from subluxating posteriorly.
IMPLICATIONS	Laxity in the posterior GH capsule, torn posterior labrum

GH = glenohumeral.

Box 13–13   Test for Posterior Instability in the Plane of the Scapula

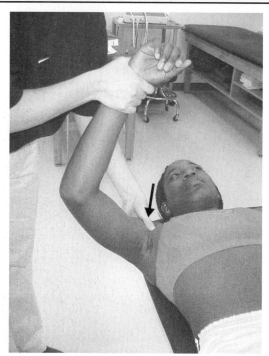

PATIENT POSITION	Lying supine The shoulder in 90° of abduction and horizontally adducted to approximately 30° to place the humerus in the plane of the scapula The elbow flexed to a comfortable position The GH joint being tested off to the side of the table
POSITION OF EXAMINER	One hand supports the weight of the arm at the elbow The opposite palm or thumb is placed over the anterior portion of the GH capsule.
EVALUATIVE PROCEDURE	Using the thumb or palm, a pressure is applied to the humeral head, attempting to drive it posteriorly on the glenoid fossa. Additional force may be used by applying a longitudinal force on the humerus by applying pressure from the elbow.
POSITIVE TEST	Pain or laxity in the posterior GH capsule or the patient displaying apprehension of a posterior subluxation
IMPLICATIONS	Laxity in the posterior GH capsule, coracohumeral ligament

GH = glenohumeral.

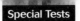
Box 13-14 Sulcus Sign for Inferior Glenohumeral Laxity

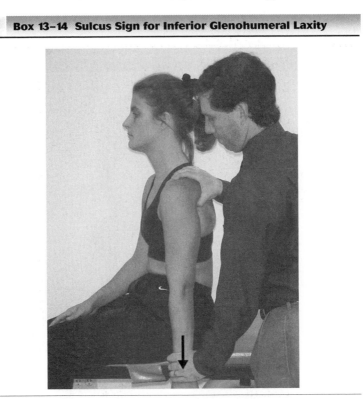

PATIENT POSITION	Sitting Arm hanging at the side
POSITION OF EXAMINER	Standing lateral to the involved side The patient's arm gripped distal to the elbow
EVALUATIVE PROCEDURE	A downward (inferior) traction force is applied to the humerus.
POSITIVE TEST	An indentation (sulcus) appears beneath the acromion process To differentiate the results of this test from those of the AC traction test for AC joint instability, the movement of the humeral head is away from the scapula and clavicle in this test. In the AC traction test, the humerus and scapula move away from the clavicle.
IMPLICATIONS	The humeral head slides inferiorly on the glenoid fossa, indicating laxity in the superior GH ligament.

AC = acromioclavicular; GH = glenohumeral.

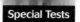

Box 13–15   The Neer Shoulder Impingement Test

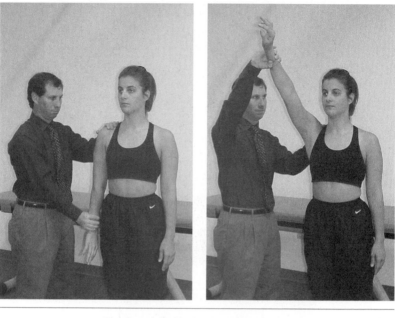

PATIENT POSITION	Standing or sitting The shoulder, elbow, and wrist in the anatomical position
POSITION OF EXAMINER	Standing lateral or forward of the involved side The patient's shoulder stabilized on the posterior aspect The examiner's other hand gripping the patient's arm distal to the elbow joint
EVALUATIVE PROCEDURE	With the elbow extended, the humerus is placed in internal rotation and the forearm is pronated. The GH joint is then forcefully moved through forward flexion as the scapula is stabilized.
POSITIVE TEST	Pain with motion, especially near the end of the ROM.
IMPLICATIONS	Pathology is present in the rotator cuff group (especially the supraspinatus) or the long head of the biceps brachii tendon. The motion of the test impinges these structures between the greater tuberosity and the inferior side of the acromion process and AC joint.

AC = acromioclavicular; GH = glenohumeral; ROM = range of motion.

Box 13-16 The Hawkins Shoulder Impingement Test

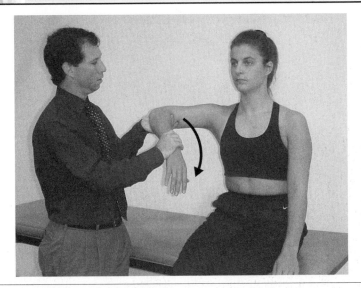

PATIENT POSITION	Sitting or standing The shoulder, elbow, and wrist in the anatomical position
POSITION OF EXAMINER	Standing lateral or forward of the involved side The examiner's other hand gripping the patient's arm at the elbow joint
EVALUATIVE PROCEDURE	With the elbow flexed, the GH joint elevated to 90° in the scapular plane. At this point, the humerus is passively internally rotated.
POSITIVE TEST	Pain with motion, especially near the end of the ROM
IMPLICATIONS	Pathology is present in the rotator cuff group (especially the supraspinatus) or the long head of the biceps brachii tendon. The motion of the test impinges these structures between the greater tuberosity and the inferior side of the acromion process.
COMMENT	If the humerus is brought in toward the sagittal plane, the chance of eliciting a false-positive result secondary to AC joint pathology increases.

AC = acromioclavicular; GH = glenohumeral; ROM = range of motion.

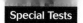

Box 13-18 Empty Can Test for Supraspinatus Pathology

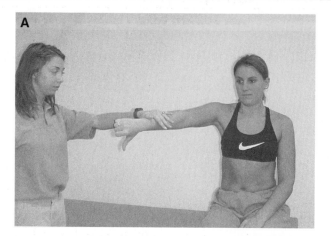

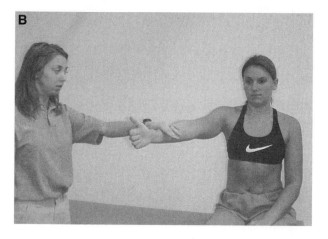

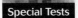

Box 13–18 Empty Can Test for Supraspinatus Pathology (Continued)	
PATIENT POSITION	Sitting or standing The GH abducted to 90° in the scapular plane, the elbow extended, and the humerus internally rotated and the forearm pronated so that the thumb points downward (internally rotated) **(A)**.
POSITION OF EXAMINER	Standing facing the patient One hand placed on the superior portion of the midforearm to resist the motion of abduction in the scapular plane
EVALUATIVE PROCEDURE	The evaluator resists abduction (applies a downward pressure).
POSITIVE TEST	Weakness or pain accompanying the movement
IMPLICATIONS	The supraspinatus tendon (1) is being impinged between the humeral head and the coracoacromial arch, (2) is inflamed, or (3) contains a lesion.
MODIFICATION	This test can be performed with the humerus externally rotated and the forearm supinated so that the thumb is facing upward, the **full can test (B)**.

GH = glenohumeral.

Shoulder and Arm

Box 13–19 Yergason's Test for Subluxation of the Biceps Tendon

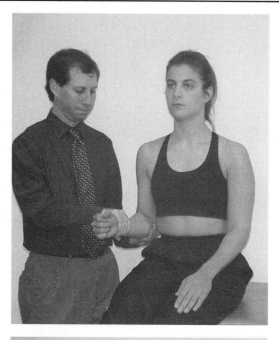

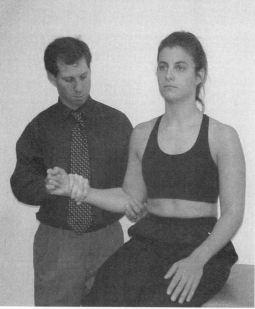

Box 13-19	**Yergason's Test for Subluxation of the Biceps Tendon** (Continued)
PATIENT POSITION	Sitting or standing GH joint in the anatomical position The elbow flexed to 90° The forearm positioned so that the lateral border of the radius faces upward (neutral position).
POSITION OF EXAMINER	Positioned lateral to the patient on the involved side The olecranon stabilized inferiorly and maintained close to the thorax The forearm stabilized proximal to the wrist
EVALUATIVE PROCEDURE	The patient provides resistance while the examiner concurrently moves the GH joint into external rotation and the proximal radioulnar joint into supination.
POSITIVE TEST	Pain or snapping (or both) in the bicipital groove
IMPLICATIONS	**Primary:** snapping or popping in the bicipital groove indicates a tear or laxity of the transverse humeral ligament. This pathology prevents the ligament from securing the long head of the tendon in its groove. **Secondary:** pain with no associated popping in the bicipital groove may indicate bicipital tendinitis.

GH = glenohumeral.

Shoulder and Arm

Box 13–20 Speed's Test for Long Head of the Biceps Brachii Tendinitis

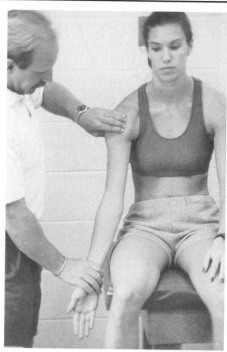

PATIENT POSITION	Sitting or standing The elbow extended The GH joint in neutral position or slightly extended to stretch the biceps brachii
POSITION OF EXAMINER	Standing lateral to and in front of the involved limb The fingers of one hand positioned over the bicipital groove while stabilizing the shoulder The forearm stabilized proximal to the wrist
EVALUATIVE PROCEDURE	The clinician resists flexion of the GH joint and elbow while palpating for tenderness over the bicipital groove.
POSITIVE TEST	Pain along the long head of the biceps brachii tendon, especially in the bicipital groove
IMPLICATIONS	Inflammation of the long head of the biceps tendon as it passes through the bicipital groove Possible tear of the transverse humeral ligament with concurrent instability of the long head of the biceps tendon as it passes through the bicipital groove

GH = glenohumeral.

Box 13-21 Ludington's Test for Biceps Brachii Pathology

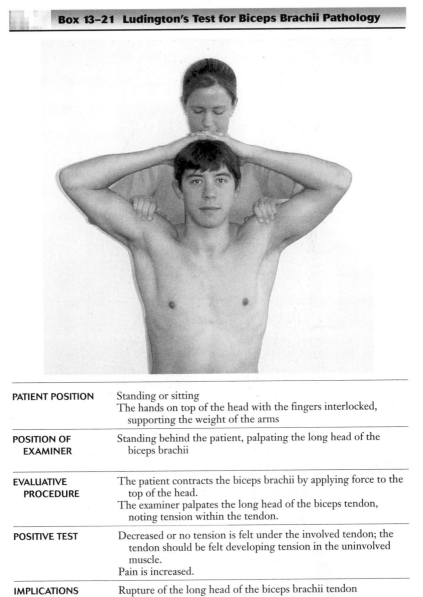

PATIENT POSITION	Standing or sitting The hands on top of the head with the fingers interlocked, supporting the weight of the arms
POSITION OF EXAMINER	Standing behind the patient, palpating the long head of the biceps brachii
EVALUATIVE PROCEDURE	The patient contracts the biceps brachii by applying force to the top of the head. The examiner palpates the long head of the biceps tendon, noting tension within the tendon.
POSITIVE TEST	Decreased or no tension is felt under the involved tendon; the tendon should be felt developing tension in the uninvolved muscle. Pain is increased.
IMPLICATIONS	Rupture of the long head of the biceps brachii tendon

Box 13-22 Active Compression Test (O'Brien's Test)

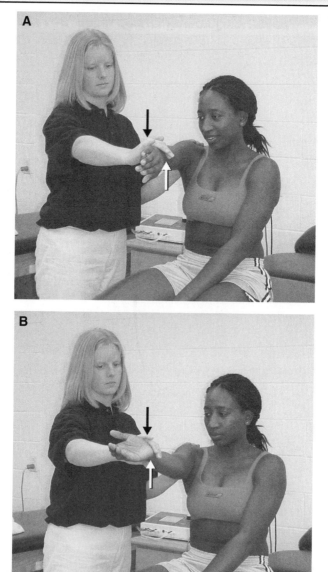

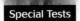

	Box 13-22 Active Compression Test (O'Brien's Test) (Continued)
PATIENT POSITION	Standing The GH joint is flexed to 90° and horizontally adducted 15° from the sagittal plane. The humerus in full internal rotation and the forearm pronated **(A)**.
POSITION OF EXAMINER	In front of the patient One hand placed over the superior aspect of the patient's distal forearm
EVALUATIVE PROCEDURE	The patient resists the examiner's downward force. The test is repeated with the humerus externally rotated and the forearm supinated **(B)**.
POSITIVE TEST	Pain that is experienced with the arm internally rotated but is decreased during external rotation: **1.** Pain or clicking within the GH joint may indicate a labral tear. **2.** Pain at the AC joint may indicate AC joint pathology.
IMPLICATIONS	SLAP lesion
COMMENTS	The presence of rotator cuff pathology may produce false-positive results.

AC = acromioclavicular; GH = glenohumeral; SLAP = superior labrum anterior to posterior tear.

Shoulder and Arm

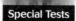

Box 13–23   Adson's Test for Thoracic Outlet Syndrome

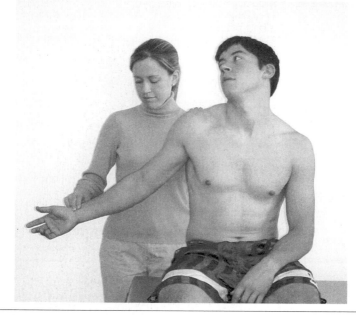

PATIENT POSITION	Sitting The shoulder abducted to 30° The elbow extended with the thumb pointing upward The humerus externally rotated
POSITION OF EXAMINER	Standing behind the patient One hand positioned so that the radial pulse is palpable
EVALUATIVE PROCEDURE	While still maintaining a feel for the radial pulse, the examiner externally rotates and extends the patient's shoulder while the face is rotated toward the involved side and extends the neck. The patient is instructed to inhale deeply and hold the breath.
POSITIVE TEST	The radial pulse disappears or markedly diminishes.
IMPLICATIONS	The subclavian artery is being occluded between the anterior and middle scalene muscles and the pectoralis minor.
COMMENT	This test often produces false-positive results.

Shoulder and Arm

Box 13-24 Allen's Test for Thoracic Outlet Syndrome

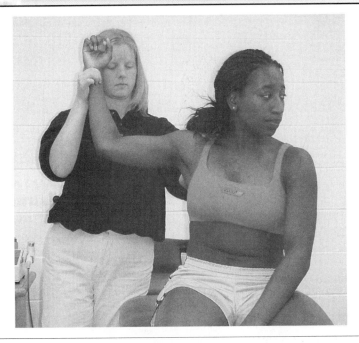

PATIENT POSITION	Sitting The head facing forward
POSITION OF EXAMINER	Standing behind the patient One hand positioned so that radial pulse is felt
EVALUATIVE PROCEDURE	The elbow is flexed to 90° while the clinician abducts the shoulder to 90°. The shoulder is then passively horizontally abducted and placed into external rotation. The patient then rotates the head towards the opposite shoulder.
POSITIVE TEST	The radial pulse disappears.
IMPLICATIONS	The pectoralis minor muscle is compressing the neurovascular bundle.
COMMENT	This test often produces false-positive results.

Box 13–25 Military Brace Position for Thoracic Outlet Syndrome

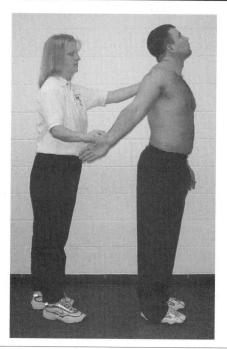

PATIENT POSITION	Standing The shoulders in a relaxed posture The head looking forward
POSITION OF EXAMINER	Standing behind the patient One hand positioned to locate the radial pulse on the involved extremity
EVALUATIVE PROCEDURE	The patient retracts and depresses the shoulders as if coming to military attention. The humerus is extended and abducted to 30°. The neck and head are hyperextended.
POSITIVE TEST	The radial pulse disappears.
IMPLICATIONS	The subclavian artery is being blocked by the costoclavicular structures of the shoulder.

Neurological Testing

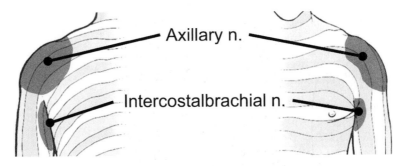

FIGURE 13-5 Neuropathies of the shoulder and upper arm. Pain may also be referred to this area from the thorax and the brachial plexus

14

The Elbow and Forearm

EVALUATION MAP: Elbow and Forearm

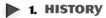 **1. HISTORY**

Location of the pain
Onset of the symptoms
Mechanism of injury
Technique
Associated sounds
Associated sensations
Previous history
General medical health

2. INSPECTION

Anterior Structures
Carrying angle
Cubital fossa

Medial Structures
Medial epicondyle
Flexor muscle mass

Lateral Structures
Alignment
Cubital recurvatum
Extensor muscle mass

Posterior Structures
Bony alignment
Olecranon process and bursa

 3. PALPATION

Anterior Structures
Biceps brachii
Cubital fossa

Brachioradialis
Wrist flexor group
Pronator quadratus

Medial Structures
Medial epicondyle
Ulna
Ulnar collateral ligament

Lateral Structures
Lateral epicondyle
Radial head
Lateral ulnar collateral ligament
Capitellum
Annular ligament
Radial collateral ligament

Posterior Structures
Olecranon process
Olecranon fossa
Triceps brachii
Anconeus
Ulnar nerve
Wrist extensors
Finger extensors
Thumb musculature

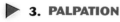 **4. RANGE OF MOTION TESTS**

Active Range of Motion
Flexion
Extension
Pronation
Supination

CHAPTER 14

Passive Range of Motion
Flexion
Extension
Pronation
Supination

Resisted Range of Motion
Flexion
Extension
Pronation
Supination

 5. LIGAMENTOUS TESTS

Valgus stress test
Varus stress test

▶ **6. NEUROLOGICAL TESTS**

Radial nerve
Medial nerve
Ulnar nerve

▶ **7. SPECIAL TESTS**

Elbow Sprains
Posterolateral rotatory instability test

Epicondylitis
Tennis elbow test

Nerve trauma
Tinel's sign

Elbow and Forearm

276   C H A P T E R 1 4   The Elbow and Forearm

History

Table 14–1	Possible Trauma Based on the Location of Pain			
	Location of Pain			
	Lateral	**Anterior**	**Medial**	**Posterior**
Soft tissue injury	Annular ligament sprain Radial collateral ligament sprain Radiocapitellar chondromalacia Lateral epicondylitis (tennis elbow) Radial nerve trauma	Biceps brachii tendinitis Rupture of the biceps brachii tendon Median nerve trauma Anterior capsule sprain	Ulnar collateral ligament sprain Medial epicondylitis Ulnar nerve trauma	Olecranon bursitis Triceps brachii tendinitis Triceps tendon rupture
Bony injury	Avulsion of the common extensor tendon Lateral epicondyle fracture Radius fracture Radial head fracture Radial head dislocation	Osteochondral fracture Avulsion of the biceps brachii tendon	Avulsion of the common flexor tendon Medial epicondyle fracture Ulna fracture Osteophyte formation	Fracture of the olecranon process

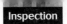
Inspection

Inspection of the Carrying Angle

Males   ## Females

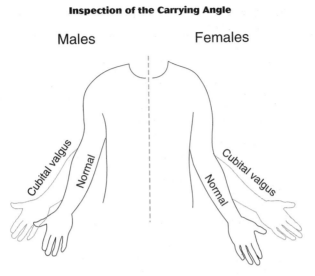

Figure 14–1 Angular relationships at the elbow. On average, women have an increased angle between the midline of the forearm and the humerus (the "carrying angle") relative to men. The normal carrying angles range from 10° to 15° for women and from 5° to 10° for men. Long-term participation in overhand throwing sports increases this angle.

PALPATION

Palpation of the Anterior Structures

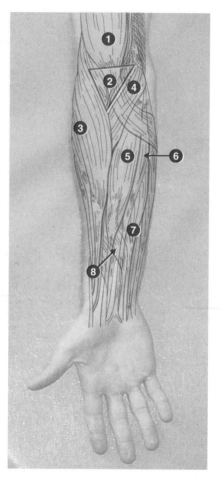

ANTERIOR STRUCTURES

1 Biceps brachii
2 Cubital fossa
3 Brachioradialis
4 Pronator teres
5 Flexor carpi radialis
6 Palmaris longus
7 Flexor carpi ulnaris
8 Pronator quadratus

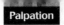
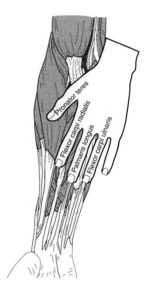

Figure 14–2 Method of approximating the superficial muscles of the flexor forearm.

Palpation of the Medial Structures

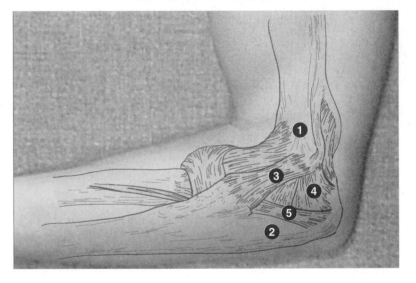

MEDIAL STRUCTURES

1 Medial epicondyle

2 Ulna

3 Ulnar collateral ligament: Anterior band

4 Ulnar collateral ligament: Posterior bundle

5 Ulnar collateral ligament: Transverse bundle

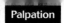
280   CHAPTER 14   The Elbow and Forearm

Palpation of the Lateral Structures

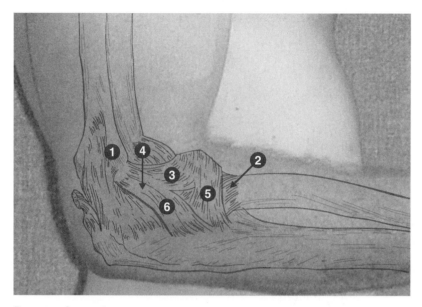

LATERAL STRUCTURES

1 Lateral epicondyle
2 Radial head
3 Radial collateral ligament
4 Capitellum
5 Annular ligament
6 Lateral ulnar collateral ligament

Palpation of the Posterior Structures

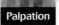

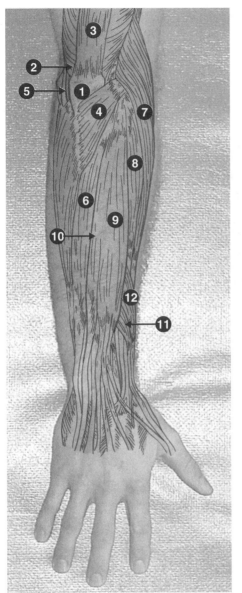

POSTERIOR STRUCTURES

1 Olecranon process
2 Olecranon fossa
3 Triceps brachii
4 Anconeus
5 Ulnar nerve
6 Extensor carpi ulnaris
7 Extensor carpi radialis brevis
8 Extensor carpi radialis longus
9 Extensor digitorum
10 Extensor digiti minimi
11 Extensor pollicis brevis
12 Abductor pollicis longus

Elbow and Forearm

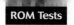
282   C H A P T E R 1 4   The Elbow and Forearm

Range of Motion Testing

Box 14–1   Elbow Goniometry

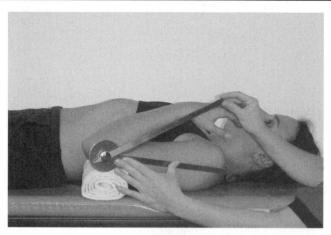

Flexion

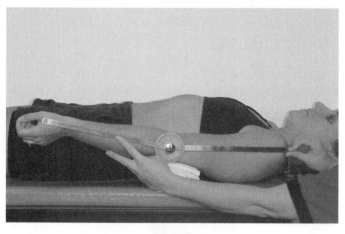

Extension

PATIENT POSITION	Supine with the humerus close to the body, the shoulder in the neutral position, and the forearm supinated
	A bolster placed under the distal humerus
GONIOMETER ALIGNMENT	
FULCRUM	Centered over the lateral epicondyle
STATIONARY ARM	Aligned with the long axis of the humerus, using the acromion process as the proximal landmark
MOVEMENT ARM	Aligned with the long axis of the radius, using the styloid process as the distal landmark.

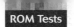

Box 14–1   **Elbow Goniometry** (Continued)

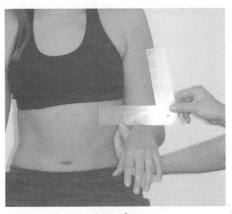

Pronation

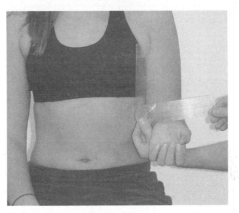

Supination

Elbow and Forearm

	Pronation	Supination
PATIENT POSITION	Sitting with the humerus held against the torso The elbow flexed to 90°	
GONIOMETER ALIGNMENT		
FULCRUM	Centered lateral to the ulnar styloid process	
STATIONARY ARM	Aligned parallel to the midline of the humerus	
MOVEMENT ARM	Across the dorsal portion of the forearm	Across the ventral portion of the forearm

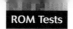

Range of Motion Testing

Table 14-2 Elbow-Capsular Patterns and End-Feels

Humeroulnar and Radiohumeral Joints
    Capsular Pattern: flexion, extension

Extension	Hard–Bony contact between the olecranon process and olecranon fossa
Flexion	Soft–Approximation between the anterior forearm and the biceps brachii
	Hard–Bony contact between the coronoid process and coronoid fossa; contact between the radial head and the radial fossa

Superior Radioulnar Joint
    Capsular Pattern: supination and pronation equally

Supination	Firm–Stretch of the radioulnar ligament; interosseous membrane; pronator teres; pronator quadratus
Pronation	Hard–Bony contact between the radius and ulna
	Firm–Stretch of the radioulnar l.; interosseous membrane; supinator; biceps brachii

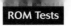
Elbow Range of Motion: Flexion and Extension

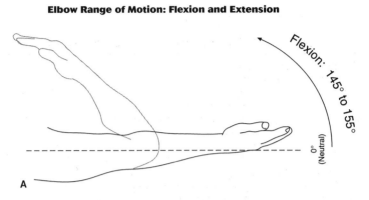

Elbow Range of Motion: Pronation and Supination

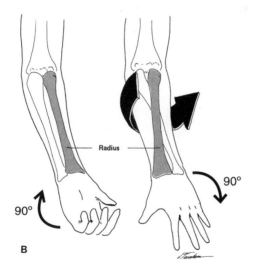

Figure 14–3 Active range of motion at the elbow. **(A)** Elbow flexion and extension; **(B)** forearm pronation and supination.

Elbow and Forearm

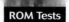
286   CHAPTER 14   **The Elbow and Forearm**

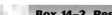

Box 14–2 Resisted Range of Motion for the Elbow

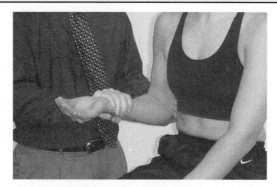

Flexion

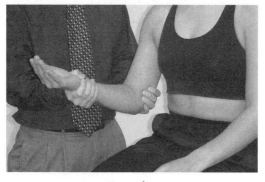

Extension

	Flexion	Extension
STARTING POSITION	Sitting or standing The shoulder in the neutral position To isolate a specific muscle during the test: Biceps brachii: forearm supinated Brachialis: forearm pronated Brachioradialis: forearm neutral	Sitting or standing The shoulder in the neutral position The forearm supinated
STABILIZATION	Anterior humerus, being careful not to compress the involved muscles	Posterior humerus, being careful not to compress the involved muscles
RESISTANCE	Over the distal forearm	Over the posterior aspect of the distal forearm
MUSCLES TESTED	See forearm position	Triceps brachii, anconeus

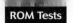
Box 14-2 Resisted Range of Motion for the Elbow (Continued)

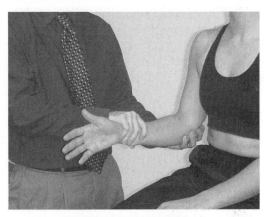

Pronation and Supination

STARTING POSITION	Seated The shoulder in the neutral position and the elbow flexed to 90° The radius facing upwards
STABILIZATION	Proximal to the elbow to prevent abduction or adduction of the glenohumeral joint
RESISTANCE	**Pronation:** resistance applied to the palmar aspect of the forearm **Supination:** resistance applied to the dorsal surface of the forearm
MUSCLES TESTED	**Pronation:** pronator quadratus, pronator teres, brachioradialis **Supination:** biceps brachii, supinator

Elbow and Forearm

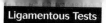

288   CHAPTER 14   The Elbow and Forearm

Ligamentous Testing

Box 14–3   Valgus Stress Test

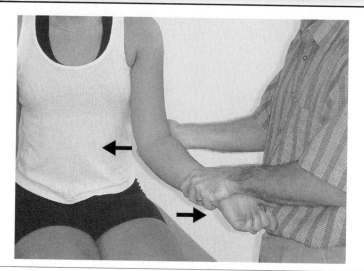

PATIENT POSITION	Standing or sitting The elbow flexed to 25°
POSITION OF EXAMINER	Standing lateral to the joint being tested One hand supporting the lateral elbow with the fingers reaching behind the joint to palpate the medial joint line with the opposite hand grasping the distal forearm
EVALUATIVE PROCEDURE	A valgus force is applied to the joint. The procedure is repeated with the elbow in various degrees of flexion.
POSITIVE TEST	Increased laxity compared with the opposite side, or pain, or both
IMPLICATIONS	Sprain of the ulnar collateral ligament, especially the anterior oblique portion. Laxity beyond 60° of flexion also implicates involvement of the posterior oblique fibers.
COMMENT	Laxity may also indicate epiphyseal injury.

Elbow and Forearm

Box 14–4 Varus Stress Test

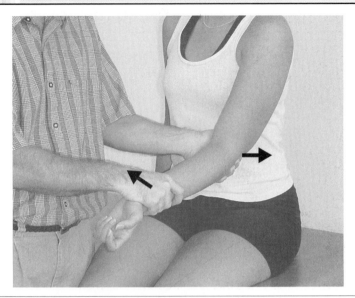

PATIENT POSITION	Standing or sitting The elbow flexed to 25°
POSITION OF EXAMINER	Standing medial to the joint being tested One hand supporting the medial elbow with the fingers reaching behind the joint to palpate the lateral joint line with the opposite hand grasping the distal forearm
EVALUATIVE PROCEDURE	A varus force is applied to the elbow. This process is repeated with the joint in various degrees of flexion.
POSITIVE TEST	Increased laxity compared with the opposite side, and/or pain is produced.
IMPLICATIONS	Moderate laxity reflects trauma to the radial collateral ligament. Gross laxity may also indicate damage to the annular or accessory lateral collateral ligament, causing the radius to displace from the ulna.
COMMENT	Laxity may also indicate epiphyseal injury.

Elbow and Forearm

SPECIAL TESTS

Box 14–5 Posterolateral Rotatory Instability Test

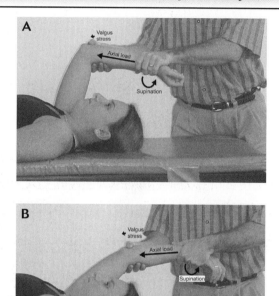

Test for posterolateral rotatory instability of the elbow consists of extending the elbow with an axial load, valgus stress, and forearm supination. The elbow subluxates as it nears full extension.

A palpable reduction may be felt as the elbow is moved back into flexion.

PATIENT POSITION	Supine The shoulder and elbow flexed to 90° and the forearm is fully supinated.
POSITION OF EXAMINER	Standing at the head of the patient One hand grasping the proximal forearm with the other hand grasping the distal forearm at the wrist **(A)**.
EVALUATIVE PROCEDURE	While applying a valgus stress and axial compression, the elbow is extended and the forearm is maintained in full supination **(B)**. The elbow then can be taken back into flexion (not shown).
POSITIVE TEST	The elbow subluxates as it is extended and can be felt to relocate as it is flexed.
IMPLICATIONS	Chronic instability of the elbow

Box 14-6 Test for Lateral Epicondylitis ("Tennis Elbow" Test)

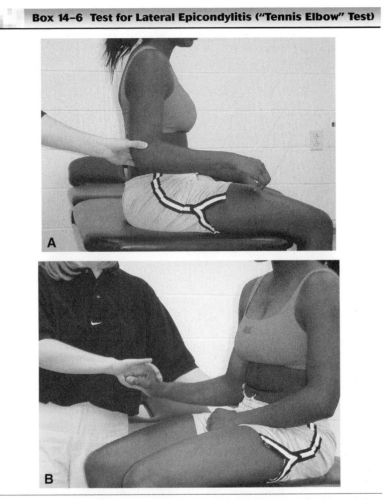

(A) The location of the thumb on the lateral epicondyle. **(B)** Resisted wrist extension.

PATIENT POSITION	Seated with the tested elbow flexed to 90°, the forearm pronated, and the fingers flexed.
POSITION OF EXAMINER	Standing lateral to the patient with one hand positioned over the dorsal aspect of the wrist and hand
EVALUATIVE PROCEDURE	The examiner resists wrist extension while palpating the lateral epicondyle and common attachment of the wrist extensors.
POSITIVE TEST	Pain in the lateral epicondyle
IMPLICATIONS	Lateral epicondylitis (tennis elbow)
MODIFICATION	This test may also be performed with the elbow in extension.

Elbow and Forearm

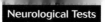

292 CHAPTER 14 The Elbow and Forearm

Neurological Testing

Nerve Distribution in the Hand

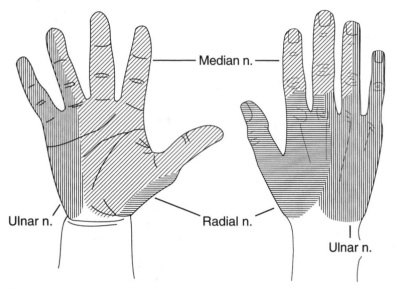

Median n.

Ulnar n.

Radial n.

Ulnar n.

FIGURE 14-4

Nerve Distribution in the Forearm

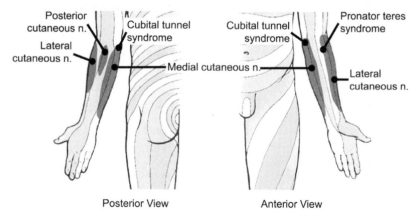

Posterior cutaneous n.

Lateral cutaneous n.

Cubital tunnel syndrome

Medial cutaneous n.

Cubital tunnel syndrome

Pronator teres syndrome

Lateral cutaneous n.

Posterior View

Anterior View

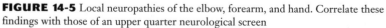

FIGURE 14-5 Local neuropathies of the elbow, forearm, and hand. Correlate these findings with those of an upper quarter neurological screen

15

The Wrist, Hand, and Fingers

EVALUATION MAP:
Wrist and Hand

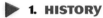 **1. HISTORY**

Location of pain
Mechanism of injury
Relevant sounds
Relevant sensation
Duration of symptoms
Description of symptoms
Previous history
General medical health

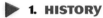 **2. INSPECTION**

General
Posture of the hand
Gross deformity
Palmar creases
Areas of cuts or scars

Wrist and Hand
Continuity of the distal radius and
    ulna
Continuity of the carpals and
    metacarpals
Alignment of the MCP joints
Posture of the wrist and hands
Ganglion cyst

Thumb and Fingers
Skin and fingernails
    Subungual hematoma
    Felon
    Paronychia
Alignment of fingernails
Finger deformities

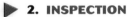 **3. PALPATION**

Palpation of the Hand
Metacarpals
MCP collateral ligaments
Phalanges
IP collateral ligaments
Thenar compartment
Thenar webspace
Central compartment
Hypothenar compartment
Ulna
    Ulnar styloid process
    Ulnar collateral ligament
Radius
    Radial styloid process
    Lister's tubercle
    Radial collateral ligament

Palpation of the Carpals
Scaphoid
Trapezium
Lunate
Pisiform
Hamate
Capitate
Trapezoid

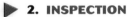 **4. RANGE OF MOTION
    TESTS**

Wrist
AROM
PROM

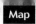

RROM
    Flexion
    Extension
    Radial deviation
    Ulnar deviation

Thumb–CMC
AROM
PROM
RROM
    Flexion
    Extension
    Abduction
    Adduction
    Opposition

Fingers
AROM
PROM
RROM
    Flexion–MCP
    Extension–MCP
    Abduction–MCP
    Adduction–MCP
    Flexion–IP joints

    Extension–IP joints
    Grip dynamometry

▶ 5. LIGAMENTOUS TESTS

Valgus stress testing–radiocarpal joint
Varus stress testing–radiocarpal joint
Glide testing of the wrist
Valgus stress testing–IP joints
Varus stress testing–IP joints
Ulnar collateral ligament– thumb

▶ 6. NEUROLOGICAL TESTS

Radial nerve
Median nerve
Ulnar nerve

▶ 7. SPECIAL TESTS

Carpal Tunnel Syndrome
Phalen's test

DeQuervain's Syndrome
Finkelstein test

AROM = active range of motion: CMC = carpometacarpal; IP = interphalangeal; MCP = metacarpophalangeal; PROM = passive range of motion; RROM = resisted range of motion.

Inspection

Inspection

Box 15–1 Pathological Hand and Finger Postures

Ape Hand

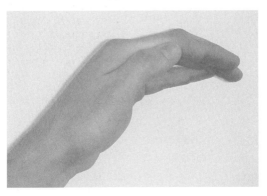

Pathology
Inhibition of the median nerve results in atrophy of the muscles within the thenar eminence. The extensor muscles draw the thumb parallel with the fingers and the patient's ability to flex or oppose the thumb is lost.

Dupuytren's Contracture

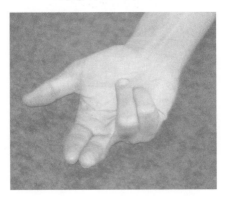

Pathology
Flexion contracture of the MCP and PIP joints is caused by a shortening or adhesion (or both) of the palmar fascia. This condition most commonly affects the 4th and 5th fingers.

MCP = metacarpophalangeal; PIP = proximal interphalangeal.

Wrist, Hand, and Fingers

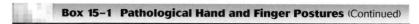

Box 15–1   Pathological Hand and Finger Postures (Continued)

Bishop's Deformity

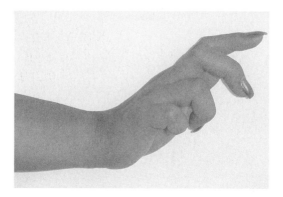

Pathology

Inhibition of the ulnar nerve results in atrophy of the hypothenar, interossei, and the medial two lumbrical muscles. The finger assumes a posture of flexion in the PIP and DIP joints that is more pronounced in the 4th and 5th fingers; also known as **"benediction deformity."**

Swan-Neck Deformity

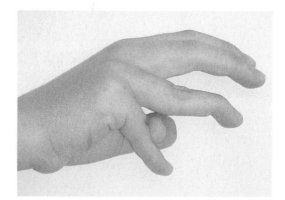

Pathology

Characterized by flexion of the MCP and DIP joints and hyperextension of the PIP joint, swan-neck deformity can be caused by a wide range of pathologies, including volar plate injuries, malunion fractures of the middle phalanx, trauma to the finger flexor or extensor muscles, or rheumatoid arthritis.

DIP = distal interphalangeal; MCP = metacarpophalangeal; PIP = proximal interphalangeal.

Box 15–1   Pathological Hand and Finger Postures (Continued)

Claw Hand

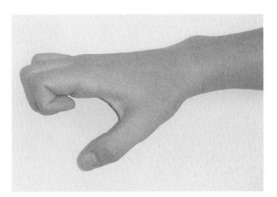

Pathology

Extension of the MCP joint and flexion of the PIP and DIP joints as the result of pathology of the ulnar and median nerve.

Volkmann's Ischemic Contracure

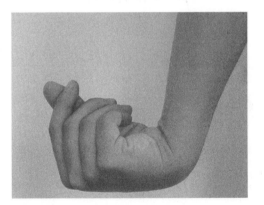

Pathology

A decrease in the blood supply to the forearm muscles can result in a flexion contracture of the wrist and fingers **(claw fingers)**. Volkmann's contracture can occur after a forearm fracture, fracture or dislocation of the elbow, or forearm compartment syndrome.

DIP = distal interphalangeal; MCP = metacarpophalangeal; PIP = proximal interphalangeal.

Wrist, Hand, and Fingers

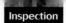
Box 15–2 Acute Finger Pathologies

Jersey Finger

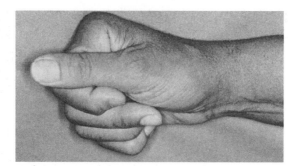

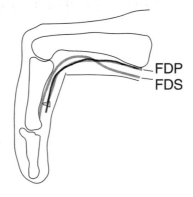

FDP
FDS

Pathology
Avulsion of the flexor digitorum profundus tendon
Posture
Inability to actively flex the DIP joint.

DIP = distal interphalangeal.

Box 15–2 Acute Finger Pathologies (Continued)

Mallet Finger

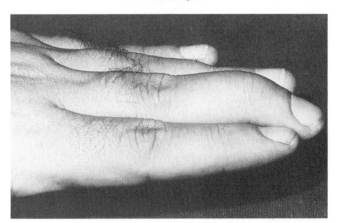

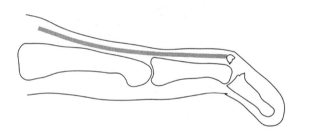

Pathology
Avulsion of the extensor digitorum longus tendon

Posture
Inability to actively extend the distal phalanx, which assumes the posture of 25° to 35° of flexion

Box 15–2 Acute Finger Pathologies (Continued)

Boutonnière Deformity

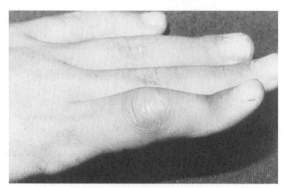

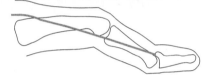

Boutonnière Deformity

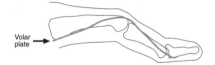

Volar
plate →

Pseudo-Boutonnière Deformity

Pathology
Boutonnière deformity: a rupture of the central extensor tendon
Pseudo-Boutonnière deformity: a rupture of the volar plate

Posture
Extension of the MCP and DIP joints and flexion of the PIP joint; acutely, the PIP joint
can be actively extended in those with boutonnière deformities but cannot be actively
extended in those with pseudo-Boutonnière deformities

DIP = distal interphalangeal; MCP = metacarpophalangeal; PIP = proximal interphalangeal.

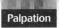
PALPATION

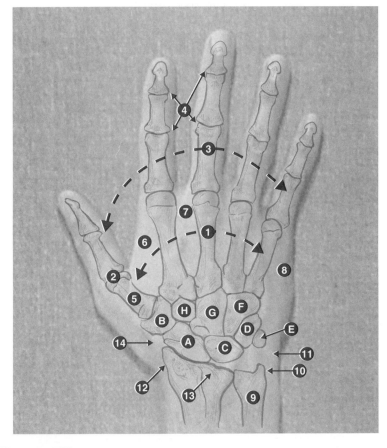

WRIST AND HAND

1 Metacarpals
2 Collateral ligaments–MCP joints
3 Phalanges
4 Collateral ligaments–IP joints
5 Thenar compartment
6 Thenar webspace
7 Central compartment

8 Hypothenar compartment
9 Ulna
10 Ulnar styloid process
11 Ulnar collateral ligament
12 Distal radius and styloid process
13 Lister's tubercle
14 Radial collateral ligament

CARPALS

A Scaphoid
B Trapezium
C Lunate
D Triquetrum

E Pisiform
F Hamate
G Capitate
H Trapezoid

302 CHAPTER 15 The Wrist, Hand, and Fingers

Range of Motion Testing

Box 15–3 Goniometry: Wrist

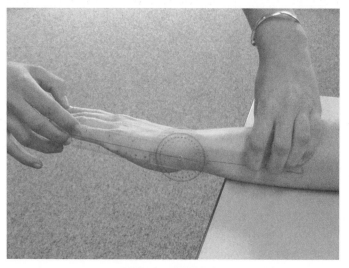

Flexion and Extension

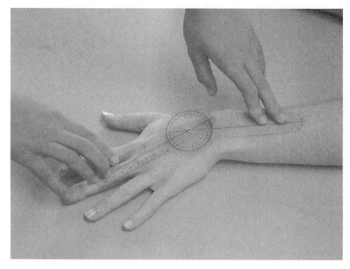

Radial and Ulnar Deviation

Box 15–3 Goniometry: Wrist

	Flexion and Extension	**Radial and Ulnar Deviation**
PATIENT POSITION	Forearm is pronated with the hand off the edge of the table. During wrist flexion, the fingers are allowed to extend. During wrist extension, the fingers are allowed to flex.	Forearm is pronated with the hand resting on the table
GONIOMETER PLACEMENT		
FULCRUM	Over the lateral joint line of the wrist	Aligned with the center of the distal radioulnar joint, just proximal to the capitate
STATIONARY ARM	Centered on the midline of the ulnar shaft	Centered over the midline of the forearm
MOVEMENT ARM	Centered on the midline of the fifth metacarpal	Centered over the third metacarpal

Wrist, Hand, and Fingers

Wrist Range of Motion: Flexion/Extension

(A)

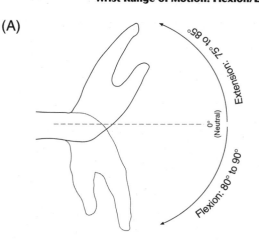

Wrist Range of Motion: Redial and Ulnar Deviation

(B)

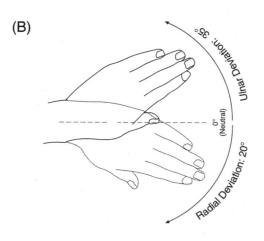

Figure 15-1 (A) Active range of motion for wrist flexion and extension. **(B)** Active range of motion for radial and ulnar deviation of the wrist

Table 15-1 Wrist-Capsular Patterns and End-Feels

Capsular Pattern: flexion and extension equally

Flexion	Firm–Stretch of the dorsal radiocarpal 1.; dorsal joint capsule
Extension	Firm–Stretch of the palmar radiocarpal 1.; palmar joint capsule
	Hard–Bony contact between the carpals and radius
Radial Deviation	Hard–Bony contact between the scaphoid and radial styloid process
	Firm–Stretch of the ulnar collateral 1.; ulnocarpal 1.
Ulnar Deviation	Firm–Stretch of the radial collateral 1.

Wrist, Hand, and Fingers

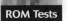

Table 15–2 Hand and Fingers-Capsular Patterns and End-Feels	

Midcarpal Joints
    Capsular Pattern: Flexion and extension equally
Metacarpophalangeal Joints
    Capsular Pattern: Flexion, extension
Fingers II–V
    Capsular Pattern: Equal limitations in all directions
Interphalangeal Joints
    Capsular Pattern: Flexion, extension

MCP Extension	Firm–Tension in the palmar joint capsule; palmar ligament
MCP Flexion	Hard–Bony contact between the phalanx and the metacarpal Firm–Stretch of the dorsal joint capsule; collateral ligaments
MCP Abduction	Firm–Stretch of the collateral ligaments; web space; palmar interossei
PIP Flexion	Hard–Bony contact between the phalanx and the metacarpal Firm–Stretch of the dorsal joint capsule; collateral ligament
PIP Extension	Firm–Tension in the palmar joint capsule; palmar ligament
DIP Flexion	Firm–Stretch of the dorsal joint capsule; collateral ligaments
DIP Extension	Firm–Tension in the palmar joint capsule; palmar ligament

Carpometacarpal Joints
    Capsular Pattern: Thumb: Abduction, extension

Flexion	Soft–Contact between the thenar eminence and palm Firm–Stretch of the dorsal joint capsule; extensor pollicis brevis; abductor pollicis brevis
Extension	Firm–Stretch of the anterior joint capsule; flexor pollicis brevis; abductor pollicis; opponens pollicis
Abduction	Firm–Stretch of the web space and fascia between the thumb and index finger, adductor pollicis; first dorsal interossei
Adduction	Soft–Contact between the thenar eminence and palm

First Metacarpophalangeal Joint
    Capsular pattern: Flexion, extension

Flexion	Hard–Bony contact between the phalanx and the metacarpal Firm–Stretch of the dorsal joint capsule; collateral ligaments; extensor pollicis brevis
Extension	Firm–Tension in the palmar joint capsule; palmar ligament; flexor pollicis brevis

Thumb Range of Motion

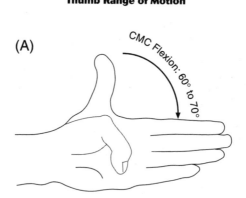

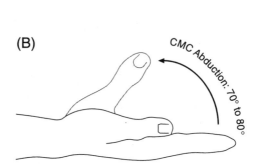

Figure 15–2 Active range of motion of the first carpometacarpal joint: **(A)** flexion; **(B)** abduction.

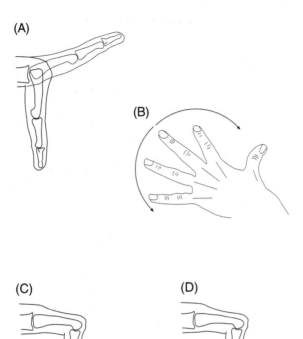

Figure 15–3 Illustration of finger range of motion: **(A)** metacarpophalangeal flexion and extension; **(B)** metacarpophalangeal abduction; **(C)** flexion of the proximal interphalangeal joint; **(D)** flexion of the proximal and distal interphalangeal joints.

Box 15–4 Goniometry: Finger

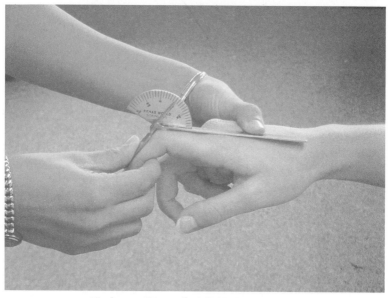

Flexion and Extension (MCP, PIP, and DIP)

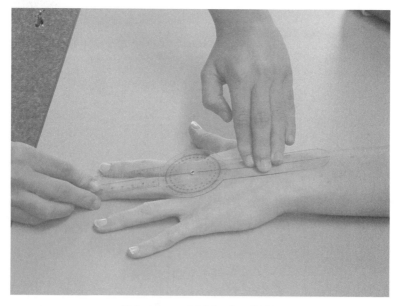

Abduction and Adduction (MCP)

Wrist, Hand, and Fingers

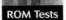

Box 15-4 **Goniometry: Finger** (Continued)

	Flexion and Extension	**Adbuction and Adduction**
PATIENT POSITION	The hand is placed in its neutral position.	The hand is placed in its neutral position.
GONIOMETER PLACEMENT		
FULCRUM	Positioned over the dorsal aspect of the joint being tested	The hand is in its neutral position with the fingers slightly spread
STATIONARY ARM	Centered on the midline of the bone proximal to the joint being tested	Centered over the MCP joint being tested
MOVEMENT ARM	Centered on the midline of the bone distal to the joint being tested	Centered over the proximal phalange of the joint being tested

MCP = metacarpophalangeal.

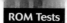

Box 15–5 Resisted Range of Motion for the Wrist	

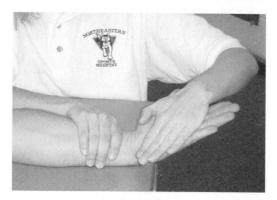

Flexion

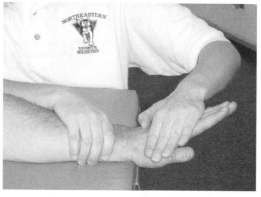

Extension

	Flexion	**Extension**
STARTING POSITION	The forearm is supinated and the wrist is extended	The forearm is pronated and the wrist is flexed
STABILIZATION	Posterior portion of the mid-forearm	Anterior portion of the mid-forearm
RESISTANCE	Palmar surface of the hand	Dorsal surface of the hand
MUSCLES TESTED	Flexor carpi radialis, flexor carpi ulnaris, flexor digitorum profundus, flexor digitorum superficialis, palmaris longus, flexor pollicis longus	Extensor carpi radialis longus, extensor carpi radialis brevis, extensor carpi ulnaris, extensor digitorum communis, extensor pollicis longus

Box 15–5 Resisted Range of Motion for the Wrist (Continued)

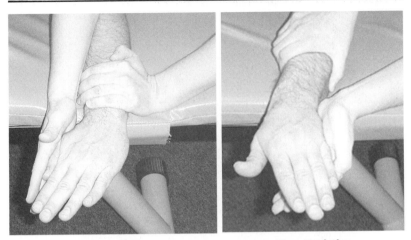

Radial Deviation	Ulnar Deviation
STARTING POSITION The forearm is supinated with the wrist in a neutral position.	The forearm is supinated with the wrist in a neutral position.
STABILIZATION Distal forearm	Distal forearm
RESISTANCE Radial side of the hand	Ulnar side of the hand
MUSCLES TESTED Extensor carpi radialis longus, extensor carpi radialis brevis, abductor pollicis longus, extensor pollicis longus, extensor pollicis brevis	Extensor carpi ulnaris, flexor carpi ulnaris

Wrist, Hand, and Fingers

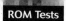

Box 15–6 Resisted Range of Motion for the First Carpometacarpal Joint

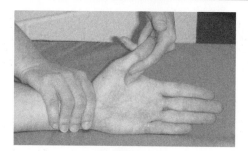

Flexion

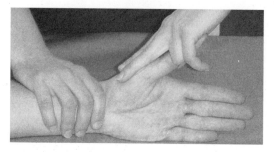

Extension

	Flexion	**Extension**
STARTING POSITION	Neutral position	Neutral position
STABILIZATION	Carpal bones	Carpal bones
RESISTANCE	Palmar aspect of the first phalanx	Dorsal aspect of the first phalanx
MUSCLES TESTED	Flexor pollicis longus, flexor pollicis brevis IP joint: flexor pollicis longus	Extensor pollicis longus, extensor pollicis brevis, abductor pollicis longus IP joint: extensor pollicis longus extensor pollicis brevis

IP = interphalangeal joint.

Box 15–6 Resisted Range of Motion for the First Carpometacarpal Joint (Continued)

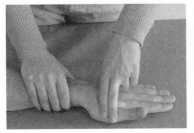 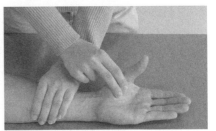

	Abduction	Adduction
STARTING POSITION	Neutral position	Neutral position
STABILIZATION	Wrist and lateral four metacarpals	Wrist and lateral four metacarpals
RESISTANCE	Lateral border of the first metacarpal	Medial border of the first metacarpal
MUSCLES TESTED	Abductor pollicis longus, abductor pollicis brevis, extensor pollicis brevis	Adductor pollicis

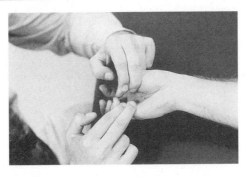

Opposition

STARTING POSITION	The thumb and fifth fingers opposed
STABILIZATION	Not applicable
RESISTANCE	The examiner attempts to separate the fingers
MUSCLES TESTED	Opponens pollicis, opponens digiti minimi

Wrist, Hand, and Fingers

Box 15–7 Resisted Range of Motion for the Fingers

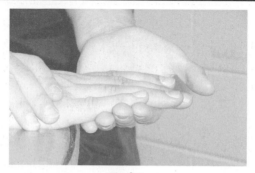

Flexion

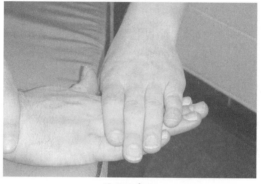

Extension

	Flexion	**Extension**
STARTING POSITION	The joint being tested is placed in the neutral position	The joint being tested is placed in the neutral position
STABILIZATION	At the joint (or joints) proximal to the joint being tested	At the joint (or joints) proximal to the joint being tested
RESISTANCE	On the palmar aspect of the phalanx distal to the joint being tested	On the dorsal aspect of the phalanx distal to the joint being tested
MUSCLES TESTED	**MCP joint:** interossei, lumbricales, flexor digitorum profundus, flexor digitorum superficialis, flexor digiti minimi (5th finger) **PIP joint:** flexor digitorum profundus, flexor digitorum superficialis **DIP joint:** flexor digitorum profundus	**MCP joint:** extensor digitorum communis **PIP and DIP joints:** extensor digitorum communis, interossei, lumbricales

DIP = distal interphalangeal; MCP = metacarpophalangeal; PIP = proximal interphalangeal.

Box 15-7 Resisted Range of Motion for the Fingers (Continued)

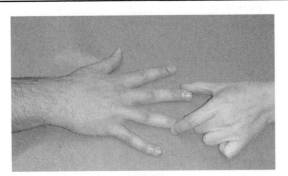

Abduction

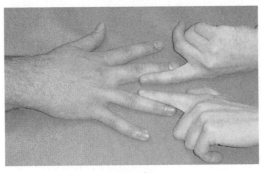

Adduction

	Abduction	Adduction
STARTING POSITION	The joint being tested is placed in the neutral position	The joint being tested is placed in the neutral position
STABILIZATION	Not applicable	Not applicable
RESISTANCE	As above	As above
MUSCLES TESTED	Dorsal interossei, abductor digiti minimi (5th finger)	Palmar interossei

Box 15–8 Grip Dynamometry

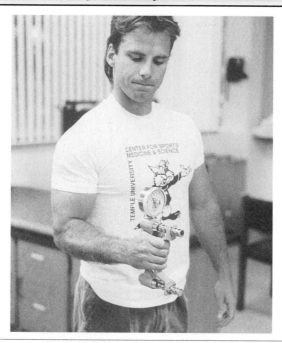

PATIENT POSITION	Holding the grip dynamometer with the elbow flexed to 90° and the radioulnar joint in its neutral position
POSITION OF EXAMINER	Standing in front of the patient, viewing the dynamometer's gauge
EVALUATIVE PROCEDURE	The dynamometer is set at one of five specified settings (1, 1.5, 2, 2.5, and 3 inches). The patient squeezes the dynamometer's handle with maximum force at every setting, with adequate recovery time allowed between bouts. The values are recorded and the test is repeated on the opposite hand.
POSITIVE TEST	Injured nondominant hand: more than 10% bilateral strength deficit compared with the dominant hand. Injured dominant hand: more than 5% bilateral strength deficit compared with the nondominant hand
IMPLICATIONS	Pathology that inhibits grip strength, the underlying cause of the weakness must be determined.
COMMENT	Because of the wide range of variation in grip strength, the outcome of each of these tests is most meaningful when compared with a baseline measure. This test can be repeated 3 times at any one setting and the results averaged.

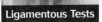
Ligamentous Tests

Box 15-9   Valgus and Varus Stress Testing of the Wrist

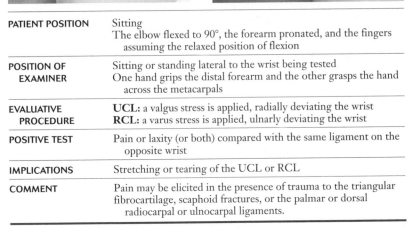

PATIENT POSITION	Sitting The elbow flexed to 90°, the forearm pronated, and the fingers assuming the relaxed position of flexion
POSITION OF EXAMINER	Sitting or standing lateral to the wrist being tested One hand grips the distal forearm and the other grasps the hand across the metacarpals
EVALUATIVE PROCEDURE	**UCL:** a valgus stress is applied, radially deviating the wrist **RCL:** a varus stress is applied, ulnarly deviating the wrist
POSITIVE TEST	Pain or laxity (or both) compared with the same ligament on the opposite wrist
IMPLICATIONS	Stretching or tearing of the UCL or RCL
COMMENT	Pain may be elicited in the presence of trauma to the triangular fibrocartilage, scaphoid fractures, or the palmar or dorsal radiocarpal or ulnocarpal ligaments.

RCL = radial collateral ligament; UCL = ulnar collateral ligament.

Wrist, Hand, and Fingers

Box 15–10 Wrist Glide Tests

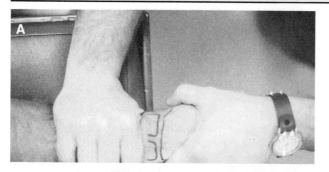

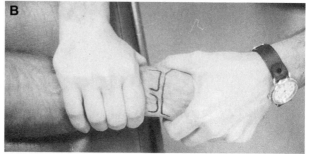

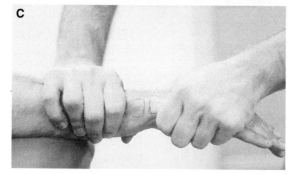

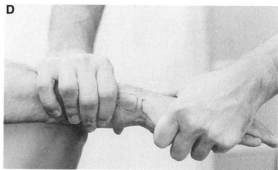

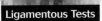
Box 15–10 Wrist Glide Tests (Continued)	

Glide testing of the wrist: radial glide **(A)**; ulnar glide **(B)**; superior glide **(C)**; and inferior glide **(D)**.

PATIENT POSITION	Sitting The elbow flexed to 90°, the forearm pronated, and the fingers assuming the relaxed position of flexion
POSITION OF EXAMINER	Sitting or standing lateral to the wrist being tested One hand grips the distal radius, and the other hand grasps the proximal carpal row.
EVALUATIVE PROCEDURE	A shear force is applied to the wrist by gliding the distal segment in a radial and ulnar direction and then in a volar and dorsal direction.
POSITIVE TEST	Pain or significant change in glide compared with the opposite side
IMPLICATIONS	Tear or stretching of the collateral or intercarpal ligaments or trauma to the triangular fibrocartilage. Decreased glide may indicate adhesions and capsular stiffness after injury or surgery.
COMMENT	This motion stresses both collateral ligaments; the determination of which ligament is involved is based on the location of pain.

Box 15–11 Valgus and Varus Testing of the Interphalangeal Joints

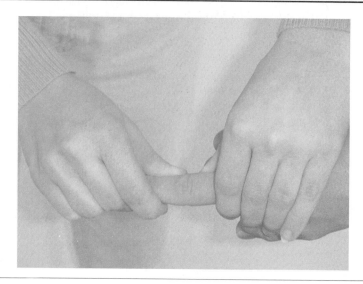

Stress testing the ulnar collateral ligament of the PIP joint. This test should be repeated using varus stress for the radial collateral ligament.

PATIENT POSITION	Sitting or standing The joint being tested is in extension.
POSITION OF EXAMINER	Standing in front of the patient, stabilizing the phalanx proximal to the joint being tested
EVALUATIVE PROCEDURE	The examiner grasps the phalanx distal to the joint being tested and applies a valgus stress to the joint. A varus stress is then applied to the joint.
POSITIVE TEST	Increased gapping, compared with the same motion on the same finger of the opposite hand Pain
IMPLICATIONS	Collateral ligament sprain
COMMENT	Except in the case of a complete disruption of the ligament, the degree of injury to the ligament cannot be established.

PIP = proximal interphalangeal.

Box 15–12 Test for Laxity of the Collateral Ligaments

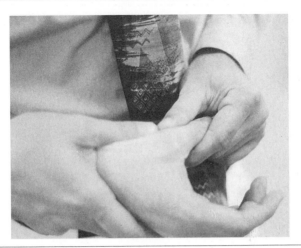

PATIENT POSITION	Sitting or standing
POSITION OF EXAMINER	Standing in front of the patient
EVALUATIVE PROCEDURE	The examiner stabilizes the first metacarpal with one hand and its proximal phalanx with the other.
	While stabilizing the first metacarpal with the thumb slightly abducted and extended, the examiner applies a valgus stress to the ulnar collateral ligament. The test is repeated with the joint in varying degrees of flexion to evaluate the dorsal capsule of the joint.
POSITIVE TEST	The ulnar side of the first metacarpophalangeal joint gaps farther than the uninjured side or the patient describes pain (or both).
IMPLICATIONS	Stretching or tearing of the ulnar collateral ligament

SPECIAL TESTS

Box 15-13 Phalen's Test for Carpal Tunnel Syndrome

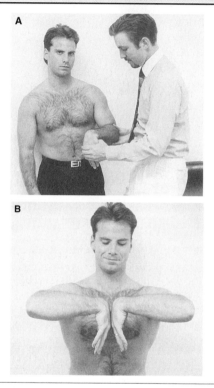

(A) Modification of Phalen's test (described below); **(B)** original test as described by Phalen.

PATIENT POSITION	Standing or seated
POSITION OF EXAMINER	Standing in front of the patient
EVALUATIVE PROCEDURE	The examiner applies overpressure during passive wrist flexion and holds the position for 1 min. This procedure is then repeated for the opposite extremity.
POSITIVE TEST	Tingling in the distribution of the median nerve distal to the carpal tunnel.
IMPLICATIONS	Median nerve compression
MODIFICATION	The traditional version of this test, in which the patient maximally flexes the wrists by pushing the dorsal aspects of the hands together, is not recommended because the patient may shrug the shoulders, causing compression of the median branch of the brachial plexus as it passes through the thoracic outlet.

Box 15–14 Finkelstein's Test for DeQuervain's Syndrome

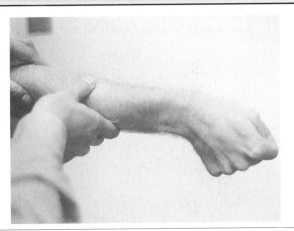

PATIENT POSITION	Seated or standing
POSITION OF EXAMINER	Standing in front of the patient
EVALUATIVE PROCEDURE	The patient tucks the thumb under the fingers by making a fist. The patient then ulnarly deviates the wrist.
POSITIVE TEST	Increased pain in the area of the radial styloid process and along the length of the extensor pollicis brevis and abductor pollicis longus tendons
IMPLICATIONS	deQuervain's syndrome (tenosynovitis of the extensor pollicis brevis and abductor pollicis longus tendons)
COMMENT	This test often produces false-positive results, so the results must be correlated with other findings of the evaluation.

Neurological Testing

Nerve Distribution in the Hand

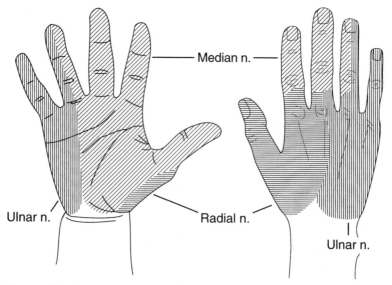

Figure 15–4 Nerve distribution in the hand.

Neurological Symptoms in the Hand

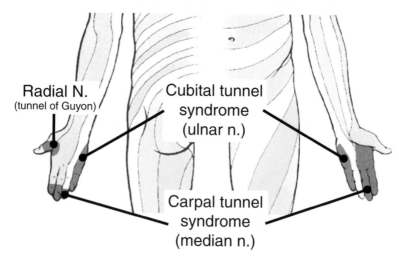

Figure 15–5 Local neuropathies of the hand. Correlate these findings with those of an upper quarter neurological screen

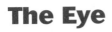

The Eye

History

Table 16–1   Mechanism of Injury and the Resulting Eye Pathology*

Size Relative to the Orbit	Elastic Property	Resulting Pathology
Larger	Hard	Orbital fracture, periorbital contusion
Larger	Elastic	Blow-out fracture, ruptured globe, corneal abrasion, traumatic iritis, periorbital contusion
Smaller	Hard	Ruptured globe, corneal abrasion, corneal laceration, traumatic iritis
Smaller	Elastic	Ruptured globe, blow-out fracture, corneal abrasion, traumatic iritis

* All of these mechanisms of injury can result in subconjunctival hemorrhage and retinal pathology.

Table 16–2   Findings Sufficient for an Immediate Referral to an Ophthalmologist

History	Inspection	Palpation	Functional Tests	Neurological Tests
Loss of all or part of the visual field	Foreign body protruding into the eye	Crepitus of the orbital rim	Restricted eye movement	Numbness over the lateral nose and cheek
Persistent blurred vision	Laceration involving the margin of the eyelid		Double vision occurring with eye movement	Pupillary reaction abnormality
Diplopia	Deep laceration of the lid			
Photophobia	Inability to open the eyelid because of swelling			
Throbbing or penetrating pain around or within the eye	Protrusion of the globe (or other obvious displacement)			
Description of mechanism for a ruptured globe	Injected conjunctiva with a small pupil			
Air escaping from the eyelid or pain when blowing the nose	Loss of corneal clarity			
	Hyphema			
	Pupillary distortion			
	Unilateral pupillary dilation or constriction			

Inspection

Eyelid Laceration

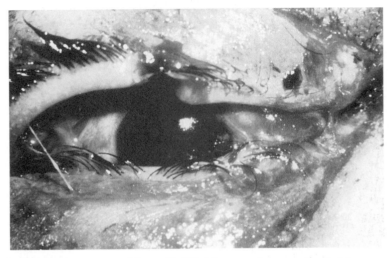

Figure 16-1 Laceration of the eyelid. This injury may also conceal underlying eye trauma.

Hyphema

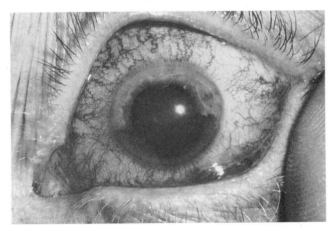

Figure 16-2 Hyphema, a collection of blood within the anterior chamber of the eye.

Subconjunctival Hemorrhage

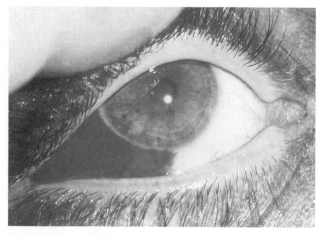

Figure 16-3 Subconjuctival hemorrhage. This condition by itself is usually benign but may conceal underlying pathology.

Teardrop Pupil

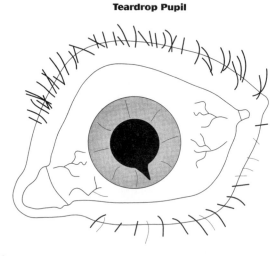

Figure 16-4 Teardrop pupil. This condition, or any other deviation in the normally round shape of the pupil, indicates serious underlying pathology such as a corneal laceration or ruptured globe.

Blowout Fracture

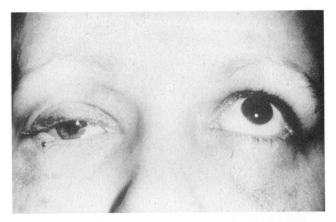

Figure 16-5 Restriction of eye motion following a blowout fracture of the orbital floor. The person's right eye is unable to gaze upward, indicating an entrapment of the inferior rectus muscle.

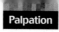
PALPATION

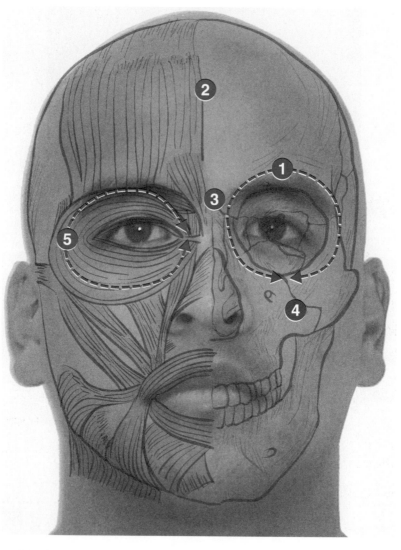

1　Orbital margin
2　Frontal bone
3　Nasal bone
4　Zygomatic bone
5　Periorbital soft tissue

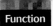

Box 16–1　Pupillary Reaction Test

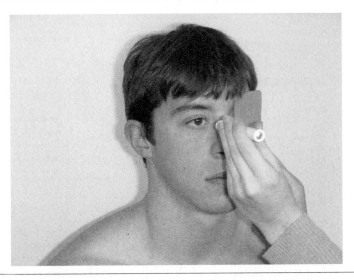

Checking for normal pupil reaction to light. If a penlight is not available, the eye tested can be covered and the pupil observed for constriction when the eye is exposed to light.

PATIENT POSITION	Sitting or standing
POSITION OF EXAMINER	Standing in front of the patient
EVALUATIVE PROCEDURE	A card, an occluder, or the patient's hand is held in front of the eye not being tested. A penlight is used to shine light into the pupil for 1 s and then removed. The examiner observes for the pupil constricting when the light is applied and dilating when the light is removed. This process is repeated for the opposite eye.
POSITIVE TEST	A pupil that is unresponsive to light or reacts sluggishly compared with the opposite eye
IMPLICATIONS	A mechanical or neurological deficit of the iris

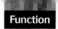

Box 16–2 Test for Eye Motility

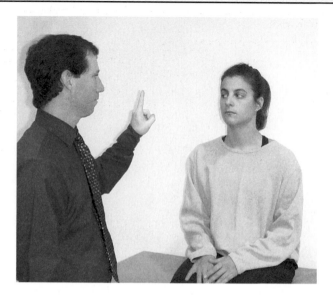

Field of gaze for eye motility

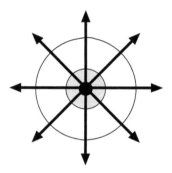

Box 16-2 Test for Eye Motility (Continued)

Checking the range of motion, motility, of the eye. The eyes should track smoothly and travel an equal distance.

PATIENT POSITION	Sitting or standing
POSITION OF EXAMINER	Standing in front of the patient, holding a finger approximately 2 ft from the patient's nose
EVALUATIVE PROCEDURE	The patient focuses on the examiner's finger. Patient is instructed to report any double vision experienced during test. The examiner moves the finger upward, downward, left, and right relative to the starting point. The patient follows this motion using only the eyes and is allowed to fix the gaze at the terminal end of each movement. The finger is then moved through the diagonal fields of gaze.
POSITIVE TEST	Asymmetrical tracking of the eyes or double vision produced at the end of the ROM.
IMPLICATIONS	Decreased motility of the eyes

ROM = range of motion.

Box 16–3 Fluorescent Dye Test for Corneal Abrasions

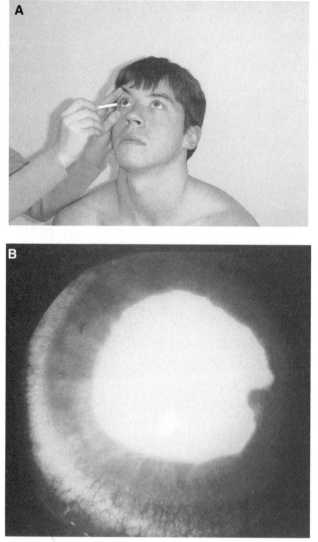

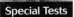

Box 16–3   Fluorescent Dye Test for Corneal Abrasions (Continued)

(A) A fluorescein strip is lightly touched to the conjunctiva. (B) A cobalt-blue light is shined into the eye to highlight the abraded area.

PATIENT POSITION	Seated or supine
POSITION OF EXAMINER	Standing in front of or beside the patient
EVALUATIVE PROCEDURE	Soak the fluorescein strip with sterile saline solution Lightly touch the wet fluorescein strip to the conjunctiva of the lower eyelid for a few seconds. Avoid placing the strip directly on the cornea. Ask the patient to blink the eye a few times to spread the solution. Darken the room and use a cobalt blue light to illuminate the eye.
POSITIVE TEST	When viewed with the cobalt blue light, corneal abrasions appear as a bright yellow-green pattern on the eye.
IMPLICATIONS	A corneal abrasion

17

The Face and Related Structures

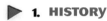 **1. HISTORY**

Location of the pain
Onset
Activity
Injury mechanism
Other symptoms

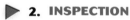 **2. INSPECTION**

Ear
Auricle
Tympanic membrane
Periauricular area

Nose
Alignment
Epistaxis
Septum and mucosa
Saddle nose deformity

Face and Jaw
Bleeding
Ecchymosis
Symmetry
Muscle tone

Oral Cavity
Lips
Teeth
Tongue
Lingual frenulum

Gums

Throat
Thyroid cartilage
Cricoid cartilage

▶ **3. PALPATION**

Nasal bone
Nasal cartilage
Zygoma
Maxilla
Temporomandibular joint
Periauricular area
External ear
Teeth
Mandible
Hyoid bone
Cartilages

▶ **4. FUNCTIONAL TESTS**

Ear
Hearing
Balance

Nose
Smell

Jaw and throat
TMJ function
Respiration

336

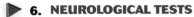

▶ 5. LIGAMENTOUS TESTS

Not applicable

▶ 6. NEUROLOGICAL TESTS

Facial muscles (CN I, II, V, VII)

Ear
Hearing (CN VIII)

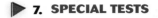

Balance (CN VIII)

Nose
Smell (CN I)

▶ 7. SPECIAL TESTS

Mandibular Fracture
Tongue blade test

CN = cranial nerve; TMJ = temporomandibular joint.

Face

Inspection

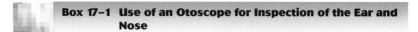

Box 17–1   Use of an Otoscope for Inspection of the Ear and Nose

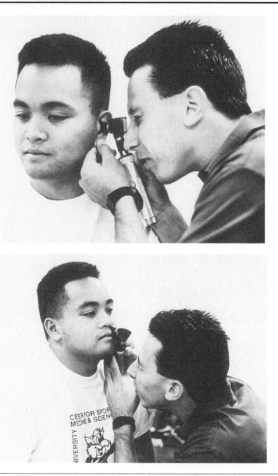

PATIENT POSITION	Seated or standing
POSITION OF EXAMINER	Position to easily access the patient's ear or nose
EVALUATIVE PROCEDURE	Use a speculum on the otoscope that will fit snugly into the opening. When inspecting the middle ear, open the auditory canal by gently pulling downward on the earlobe or upward on the apex of the external ear.

PALPATION

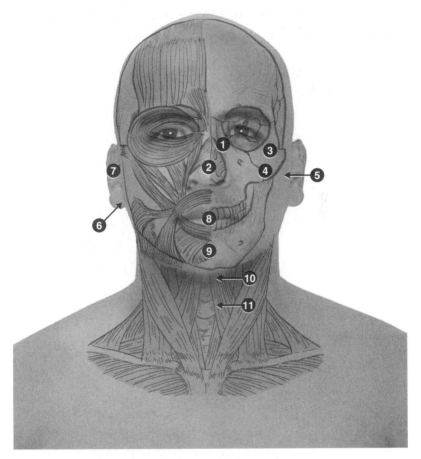

1   Nasal bone
2   Nasal cartilage
3   Zygoma
4   Maxilla
5   TMJ
6   Periauricular area
7   External ear
8   Teeth
9   Mandible
10 Hyoid bone
11 Thyroid cartilage, cricoid cartilage

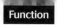
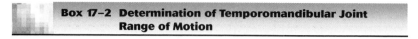

Box 17-2 Determination of Temporomandibular Joint Range of Motion

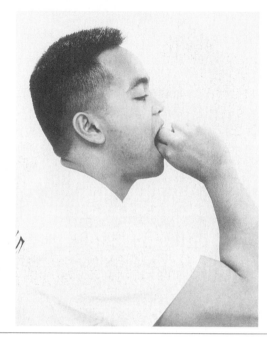

PATIENT POSITION	Seated or standing
POSITION OF EXAMINER	In front of the patient
EVALUATIVE PROCEDURE	The patient attempts to place as many flexed knuckles as possible between the upper and lower teeth.
POSITIVE TEST	The patient is unable to place a minimum of two knuckles within the mouth.
IMPLICATIONS	Decreased TMJ ROM

ROM = range of motion; TMJ = temporomandibular joint.

Box 17-3 Tongue Blade Test

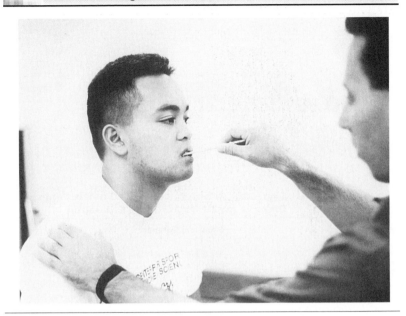

PATIENT POSITION	Seated
POSITION OF EXAMINER	Standing in front of the patient
EVALUATIVE PROCEDURE	A tongue blade (tongue depressor) is placed in the patient's mouth. As the patient attempts to hold the tongue blade in place, the examiner rotates (twists) the blade.
POSITIVE TEST	The patient is unable to maintain a firm bite or pain is elicited.
IMPLICATIONS	Possible mandibular fracture

18

Head and Neck Injuries

Table 18–1 Signs and Symptoms of a Head or Neck Injury to Observe for Throughout the Evaluation	
Area	Signs and Symptoms
Brain	Amnesia (retrograde and anterograde) Confusion Disorientation Irritability Incoordination Dizziness Headache
Ocular	Blurred vision Photophobia Nystagmus
Ears	Tinnitus Dizziness
Stomach	Nausea Vomiting
Systemic	Unusually fatigued

Table 18–2 Behavioral Signs and Symptoms of Concussion

Sign	Behavior
Vacant stare	Confused or blank facial expression
Delayed verbal and motor responses	Slow to answer questions or follow instructions
Inability to focus attention	Easily distracted; unable to complete normal activities
Disorientation	Walking in the wrong direction; time, date, and place disorientation
Slurred or incoherent speech	Rambling, disjointed, incomprehensible statements
Gross incoordination	Stumbling; inability to walk a straight line
Heightened emotions	Appearing distraught, crying for no apparent reason, emotional responses that are out of proportion to the circumstances
Memory deficits	As evidenced by the retrograde and anterograde memory tests

History

	Box 18-1 **Determination of Retrograde Amnesia**
PATIENT POSITION	**On-field:** In the athlete's current position **Sideline:** Standing sitting, or lying down
POSITION OF EXAMINER	In a position to hear the patient's response
EVALUATIVE PROCEDURE	The patient is asked a series of questions beginning with the time of the injury. Each successive question progresses backward in time, as described by the following set of questions: What happened? What play were you running? (or other applicable question regarding the patient's activity at the time of injury) Where are you? Who am I? Who are you playing? What quarter is it (or what time is it)? What did you have for a pregame meal (or what did you have to eat for lunch)? Who did you play last week?
POSITIVE TEST	The patient has difficulty remembering or cannot remember events occurring before the injury.
IMPLICATIONS	Retrograde amnesia, the severity of which is based on the relative amount of memory loss demonstrated by the inability to recall events Not remembering events from the day before is more significant than not remembering more recent events The same set of questions should be repeated to determine whether the memory is returning, deteriorating, or remaining the same. Further deterioration of the memory or acutely profound memory loss that does not return in a matter of minutes warrants the immediate termination of the evaluation and transportation to an emergency medical facility.
COMMENT	Record the patient's response and verify the answers with the athlete's teammates or coach.

Box 18–2	**Determination of Anterograde Amnesia**
PATIENT POSITION	Sitting or lying
POSITION OF EXAMINER	In a position to hear the patient's response
EVALUATIVE PROCEDURE	The athlete is given a list of four unrelated items with instructions to memorize them, for example: Hubcap Film Dog tags Ivy The list is immediately repeated by the patient to ensure that it has been memorized. The patient is asked to repeat the list to the examiner every 5 minutes.
POSITIVE TEST	The inability to recite the list completely
IMPLICATIONS	Anterograde amnesia, possibly the result of intracranial bleeding
COMMENT	This test is usually performed after the test for retrograde amnesia.

Box 18–3 Postures Assumed After Spinal Cord Injury

Decerebrate posture

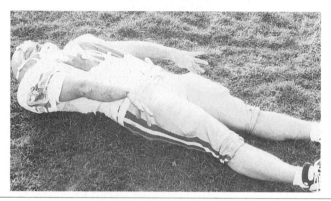

Posture
Extension of the extremities and retraction of the head

Pathology
Lesion of the brain stem; also possible secondary to heat stroke

Decorticate posture

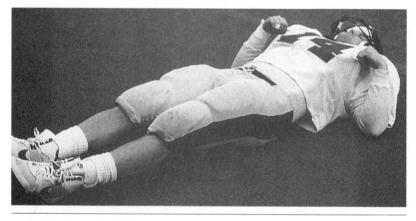

Posture
Flexion of the elbows and wrists, clenched fists, and extension of the lower extremity

Pathology
Lesion above the brain stem

Box 18–3 Postures Assumed After Spinal Cord Injury (Continued)

Flexion Contracture

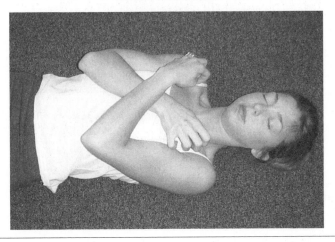

Posture
Arms flexed across the chest

Pathology
Spinal cord lesion at the C5-C6 level

Table 18–3 Inspection of Respiration

Type	Characteristics	Implications
Apneustic	Prolonged inspirations unrelieved by attempts to exhale	Trauma to the pons
Biot's	Periods of apnea followed by hyperventilation	Increased intracranial pressure
Cheyne-Stokes	Periods of apnea followed by breaths of increasing depth and frequency	Frontal lobe or brain stem trauma
Slow	Respiration consisting of fewer than 12 breaths per minute	CNS disruption
Thoracic	Respiration in which the diaphragm is inactive and breathing occurs only through expansion of the chest; normal abdominal movement is absent	Disruption of the phrenic nerve or its nerve roots

CNS = central nervous system.

Table 18-4 Inspection of Pulse

Type	Characteristics	Implication
Accelerated	Pulse > 150 beats per minute (bpm) (> 170 bpm usually has fatal results)	Pressure on the base of the brain; shock
Bounding	Pulse that quickly reaches a higher intensity than normal, then quickly disappears	Ventricular systole and reduced peripheral pressure
Deficit	Pulse in which the number of beats counted at the radial pulse is less than that counted over the heart itself	Cardiac arrhythmia
High tension	Pulse in which the force of the beat is increased; an increased amount of pressure is required to inhibit the radial pulse	Cerebral trauma
Low tension	Short, fast, faint pulse having a rapid decline	Heart failure; shock

bpm = beats per minute.

Box 18–4 Romberg's Test

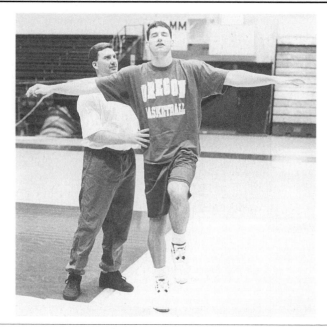

PATIENT POSITION	Standing with the feet shoulder width apart
POSITION OF EXAMINER	Standing lateral or posterior to the patient, ready to support the patient as needed
EVALUATIVE PROCEDURE	The patient shuts the eyes and abducts the arms to 90° with the elbows extended. The patient tilts the head backward and lifts one foot off the ground while attempting to maintain balance. If this portion of the examination is adequately completed, the patient is asked to touch the index finger to the nose (with the eyes remaining closed).
POSITIVE TEST	The patient displays gross unsteadiness.
IMPLICATIONS	Lack of balance and/or coordination indicating cerebellular dysfunction

Box 18–5 Tandem Walking

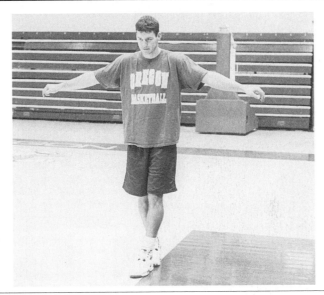

PATIENT POSITION	Standing with the feet straddling a straight line (e.g., sideline)
POSITION OF EXAMINER	Beside the patient ready to provide support
EVALUATIVE PROCEDURE	The patient walks heel-to-toe along the straight line for approximately 10 yd. The patient returns to the starting position by walking backward.
POSITIVE TEST	The patient is unable to maintain a steady balance
IMPLICATIONS	Cerebral or inner ear dysfunction that inhibits balance

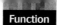

Box 18–6 Balance Error Scoring System (Bess)

Firm Surface Bout

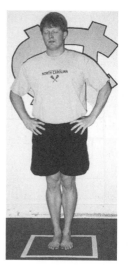 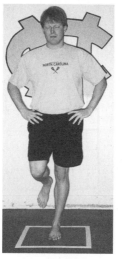 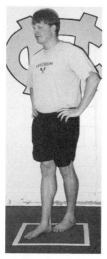

Double Leg Stance   Single Leg Stance   Tandem Leg Stance

Soft Surface Bout

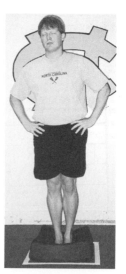 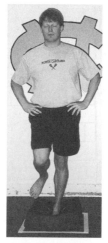 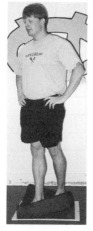

Double Leg Stance   Single Leg Stance   Tandem Leg Stance

The balance error scoring system involves three different stances, each completed twice, once while standing on a firm surface and again while standing on a foam surface.

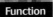
Box 18–6 Balance Error Scoring System (Bess) (Continued)	
PATIENT POSITION	The patient is barefoot or wearing socks. The ankle must not be taped during the test. The patient assumes the following stances for each phase of the test: **Phase 1:** Double leg stance **Phase 2:** Single leg stance—standing on the nondominant leg. The non—weight-bearing hip is flexed to 20° to 30° and the knee is flexed to 40° to 50°. **Phase 3:** Tandem leg stance—the nondominant leg is placed behind the dominant leg and the patient stands in a heel-toe manner. The patient's hands are placed on the iliac crests. The eyes are closed during the test.
POSITION OF EXAMINER	The examiner stands in front of the athlete. A stopwatch is required to time the trials. A second clinician acts as a spotter.
EVALUATIVE PROCEDURE	The first battery of tests is performed with the patient standing on a firm surface. The patient assumes the double leg stance and attempts to hold the position for 20 seconds. The test is repeated using the single leg stance and then the tandem leg stance. The second battery of tests is performed with the patient standing on a piece of medium density foam (60 kg/m³) that is 45 cm × 45 cm and 13 cm thick. The trial is incomplete if the patient cannot hold the testing position for a minimum of 5 seconds.
SCORING	One point is scored for each of the following errors: Lifting hands off the iliac crest Opening the eyes Stepping, stumbling, or falling Moving the hip into more than 30° of flexion or abduction Lifting the foot or heel Remaining out of the testing position for more than 5 seconds If more than one error occurs simultaneously, only one error is recorded. Patients who are unable to hold the testing position for 5 seconds are assigned the score of 10.
POSITIVE TEST	Scores that are 25% above the patient's baseline or the norm
IMPLICATIONS	Impaired cerebral function

Box 18–7 Halo Test

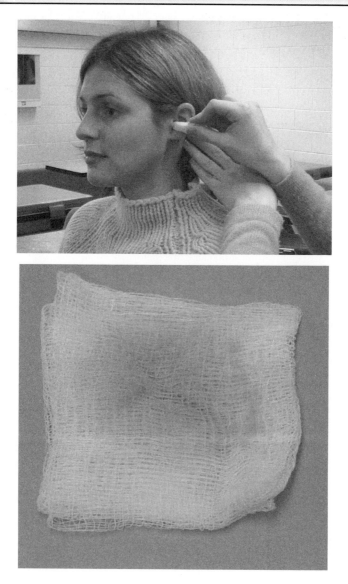

Box 18-7   Halo Test (Continued)

PATIENT POSITION	Lying or sitting
POSITION OF EXAMINER	Lateral to the patient's ear.
EVALUATIVE PROCEDURE	Fold a piece of sterile gauze into a triangle. Using the point of the gauze, collect a sample of the fluid leaking from the ear or nose and allow it to be absorbed by the gauze.
POSITIVE TEST	A pale yellow "halo" will form around the sample on the gauze.
IMPLICATIONS	Cerebrospinal fluid leakage

Box 18-8 Standardized Assessment of Concussion Tool

Orientation (1 point each)

	Correct
Month	☐
Date	☐
Day of week	☐
Year	☐
Time (within 1 hr)	☐
Score	**___/5**

Delayed Recall (1 point each)

	Correct
Word 1	☐
Word 2	☐
Word 3	☐
Word 4	☐
Word 5	☐
Score	**___/5**

Immediate Memory (1 point for each correct response)

	Trial 1	Trial 2	Trial 3
Word 1	☐	☐	☐
Word 2	☐	☐	☐
Word 3	☐	☐	☐
Word 4	☐	☐	☐
Word 5	☐	☐	☐
Score			**___/15**

Summary of total scores

Orientation	___ /5
Immediate memory	___ /15
Concentration	___ /5
Delayed recall	___ /5
TOTAL SCORE	**___ /30**

Concentration
Reverse digits (1 point each for each string length)

		Correct
3-8-2	5-1-8	☐
2-7-9-3	2-1-6-8	☐
5-1-8-6-9	9-4-1-7-5	☐
6-9-7-3-5-1	4-2-8-9-3-7	☐

Months of the year in reverse order (1point for entire sequence correct)

	Correct
Dec-Nov-Oct-Sep-Aug-Jul	
Jun-May-Apr-Mar-Feb-Jan	☐
Score	**___/5**

The following are performed between the Immediate Memory and Delayed Recall portions of the SAC, along with tests for memory, cerebral function, and strength.

Neurologic Screening
Recollection of the injury
Strength:
Sensation:
Coordination

Exertional Maneuvers (when appropriate)
1 40-yard sprint
5 sit-ups
5 push-ups
5 knee bends

Box 18-8 Standardized Assessment of Concussion Tool (Continued)

Procedures (Administration time is approximately 5 minutes): proper training is required for appropriate use.

Orientation	Patient is asked to identify the current place in time and receives 1 point for each correct response.
Immediate memory	The patient is asked to memorize a list of 5 random words. The list of words is repeated 3 times in succession, with 1 point being awarded for each correct response for a maximum total of 15 points. This list of words will be used for the delayed memory testing, but do not inform the patient as such.
Neurological screening	The patient is evaluated for loss of consciousness, amnesia, etc.
Concentration	**Reverse digits:** The patient is given a sequence of numbers and asked to repeat them in reverse order (i.e., 2-8-3 would be recited as 3-8-2). If the patient correctly responds on the first attempt, progress to the next string length. If the patient incorrectly responds on the first attempt, use a second set of digits for the second attempt. If the patient incorrectly responds on the second attempt, move on to months of the year. **Months of year:** The patient is asked to recite the months of the year in reverse order.
Delayed recall	Approximately 5 minutes following the "Immediate Memory" test, the patient is asked to recall the list of words that were used for the immediate memory test. One point is awarded for each correct response.
Total	The scores for each of the four sections are totaled to yield an overall index of impairment.

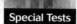

Table 18-4   The Glasgow Coma Scale

Response	Points	Action
Eye opening		
Spontaneously	4	Reticular system is intact; patient may not be aware
To verbal command	3	Opens eyes when told to do so
To pain	2	Opens eyes in response to pain
None	1	Does not open eyes to any stimuli
Verbal		
Oriented, converses	5	Relatively intact CNS; aware of self and surroundings
Disoriented, converses	4	Well articulated, organized, but disoriented
Inappropriate words	3	Random, exclamatory words
Incomprehensible	2	No recognizable words
No response	1	No audible sounds or intubated
Motor		
Obeys verbal commands	6	Readily moves limbs when told to
Localizes painful stimuli	5	Moves limb in an effort to avoid pain
Flexion withdrawal	4	Pulls away from pain with a flexion motion
Abnormal flexion	3	Exhibits decorticate rigidity
Extension	2	Exhibits decerebrate rigidity
No response	1	Demonstrates dypotonicity, flaccid: Suggests loss of medullary function or spinal cord injury

CNS = central nervous system.

Table 18-5 Cranial Nerve Function

Number	Name	Type	Function
I	Olfactory	Sensory	Smell
II	Optic	Sensory	Vision
III	Oculomotor	Motor	Effect on pupillary reaction and size Elevation of upper eyelid Eye adduction and downward rolling
IV	Trochlear	Motor	Upward eye rolling
V	Trigeminal	Mixed	Motor: muscles of mastication Sensation: nose, forehead, temple, scalp, lips, tongue, and lower jaw
VI	Abducens	Motor	Lateral eye movement
VII	Facial	Mixed	Motor: muscles of expression Sensory: taste
VIII	Vestibulocochlear	Sensory	Equilibrium Hearing
IX	Glossopharyngeal	Mixed	Motor: pharyngeal muscles Sensory: taste
X	Vagus	Mixed	Motor: muscles of pharynx and larynx Sensory: gag reflex
XI	Accessory	Motor	Trapezius and sternocleidomastoid muscles
XII	Hypoglossal	Motor	Tongue movement

Table 18-6   Concussion Rating Systems

Rating System	Signs and Symptoms		
	Grade I	**Grade II**	**Grade III**
American Academy of Neurology	No loss of consciousness Transient confusion Concussion symptoms resolve in less than 15 minutes	No loss of consciousness Transient confusion Concussion symptoms or mental status abnormalities on examination resolve in more than 15 minutes	Any loss of consciousness either brief (seconds) or prolonged (minutes).
American College of Sports Medicine Guidelines	None or transient retrograde amnesia None to slight mental confusion No loss of coordination Transient dizziness Rapid recovery	Retrograde amnesia; memory may return slight to moderate mental confusion Moderate dizziness Transitory tinnitus Slow recovery	Sustained retrograde amnesia; anterograde is possible with intracranial hemorrhage Severe mental confusion Profound loss of coordination Obvious motor impairment Prolonged tinnitus Delayed recovery
Cantu Concussion Rating Guidelines	No loss of consciousness Concussion symptoms resolving in less than 15 minutes Posttraumatic amnesia for less than 30 minutes	Loss of consciousness for less than 5 minutes Posttraumatic amnesia for more than 30 minutes but less than 24 hours	Loss of consciousness for more than 5 minutes Posttraumatic amnesia for more than 24 hours
Colorado Medical Society Concussion Rating Guidelines	No loss of consciousness Transient confusion No amnesia	No loss of consciousness Transient confusion Amnesia	Loss of consciousness

19

Environmental Injury

Environmental

Table 19–1 Signs and Symptoms of Dehydration	
Initial stages	Thirst Irritability General discomfort
Late stages	Headache Weakness Dizziness Cramps Chills Vomiting Nausea Decreased performance

Table 19–2 Rehydration Strategies	
Strategy	**Comments**
Pre-exercise hydration	Two to three hours before competition: Consume 500 to 600 mL (17 to 20 fl oz) of water or sports drink Ten to twenty minutes before competition: Consume 200 to 300 mL (7 to 10 fl oz) of water or sports drink
Hydration maintenance	Every 10 to 20 minutes: Consume 200 to 300 mL (7 to 10 fl oz) of water or sports drink Prevent the athlete from losing more than 2% of body weight through water loss
Postexercise hydration	Within 2 hours: Replace water, carbohydrates, and electrolytes lost during activity

Table 19-3 Signs and Symptoms of Heat Illness

Evaluative Finding	Heat Cramps	Heat Syncope	Heat Exhaustion	Heat Stroke
Core temperature*	WNL**	WNL	103°F or above	102°F to 104°F or above
Skin color and temperature	WNL	WNL	Cool Pale	Hot Red
Sweating	Moderate to profuse	WNL	Profuse	Slight to profuse Sweat mechanism failing
Pulse	WNL	Rapid and weak	Rapid and weak	Tachycardia
Blood pressure	WNL	A sudden, imperceptible drop in blood pressure, which rapidly returns to normal	Low	High
Respiration	WNL	WNL	Hyperventilation	Rapid
Mental state	WNL	Dizziness Fainting	Dizziness Fatigue Slight confusion	Confusion Violent behavior Unconsciousness
Other findings	Cramping in one or more muscles		Headache Nausea Vomiting Thirst	Headache Nausea Vomiting Dilated pupils Decerebrate posture

WNL = within normal limits.
* As determined by the rectal temperature.
** Within normal limits for an exercising athlete.

Enviromental

Environmental

Table 19–4 Guidelines for Modification of Athletic Competition in Hot or Humid Environments

Dry Bulb Temperature, °F	Wet Bulb Temperature, °F	Humidity, %	Consequences
80 to 90	68	<70	No extraordinary precautions are required for athletes not predisposed to heat injury. Athletes who are predisposed (e.g., unconditioned, unacclimated, or losing more than 3% of body weight from water loss) require close observation.
80 to 90 90 to 100	69 to 79	>70 <70	Regular rest breaks are necessary. Loose, breathable clothing should be worn, and wet uniforms require regular changing.
90 to 100 >100	>80	>70	Practice should be shortened and modified. The use of protective equipment covering the body should be curtailed.
	>82		Practice should be canceled

Table 19–5 Calculation of the Wind Chill Factor

Actual Thermometer Reading °F

Wind Speed, MPH	50	40	30	20	10	0	−10	−20	−30	−40	−50	−60
	Wind Chill Factor °F											
Calm	50	40	30	20	10	0	−10	−20	−30	−40	−50	−60
5	48	37	27	16	6	25	−15	−26	−36	−47	−57	−68
10	40	28	16	4	−9	−24	−33	−46	−58	−70	−83	−95
15	36	22	9	−5	−18	−32	−45	−58	−72	−85	−99	−112
20	32	18	4	−10	−25	−39	−53	−67	−82	−96	−110	−124
25	30	16	0	−15	−29	−44	−59	−74	−88	−104	−118	−133
30	28	13	−2	−18	−33	−48	−63	−79	−94	−109	−125	−140
35	27	11	−4	−20	−35	−51	−67	−82	−98	−113	−129	−145
40	26	10	−6	−21	−37	−53	−69	−85	−100	−116	−132	−148

Little danger

Moderate danger
Skin freezes within 1 min

Extreme danger
Skin freezes rapidly (< 1 min)

Environmental

Table 19-6 Evaluative Findings: Hypothermia

Segment	Finding
Onset	Gradual A cold, damp windy environment predisposes athletes to hypothermia
Pupils	Dilated in severe hypothermia
Pulse	Slow and weak
Blood pressure	Hypotension
Respiration	Shallow and irregular
Muscular function	*Slight:* Shivering *Mild:* Motor impairment *Severe:* Extreme motor impairment followed by muscle rigidity
Mental status	*Slight:* The athlete's mental focus begins to drift from the task at hand *Mild:* Desire to warm up *Severe:* Desire to sleep

20

Cardiopulmonary Conditions

EVALUATION MAP:
Cardiopulmonary Conditions

▶ **1. HISTORY**

Location of the pain
Current symptoms
Prior symptoms
Onset
Mechanism

▶ **2. INSPECTION AND**
PALPATION

Unconscious Athlete
Airway
Breathing
    Bradypnea
    Tachypnea
Circulation

Conscious Athlete
Position of the athlete

Skin color
Airway
Breathing
Circulation
Sweating
Responsiveness
Nausea and vomiting

▶ **3. VITAL SIGNS**

Pulse
Blood pressure
Respiration

▶ **4. SPECIAL TESTS**

Peak flow meter

367

History

Table 20–1 Signs and Symptoms of Cardiopulmonary Conditions

Cardiovascular	Both	Pulmonary
Panic	Chest pain	Congestion
Dizziness	Respiratory distress	Wheezing
Nausea		Fatigue
Vomiting		Anxiety
Sweating		Tingling in fingers and toes
Decreased blood pressure		Spasm in fingers and toes
Distended jugular vein		Periorbital numbness
Pallor		Pain in mid and upper posterior
Clutching at chest		thorax
Shoulder pain		
Epigastric pain		

Table 20–2 Heart Sounds

Sound	Status	Interpretation
"Lubb"	Normal systole	Ventricular contraction; synchronous with the carotid pulse
"Dupp"	Normal diastole	Closure of the aortic and pulmonary valves
Soft, blowing "lubb"	Abnormal systole	Associated with anemia or other changes in blood constituents
Loud, booming "lubb"	Abnormal systole	Aneurysm
Sloshing "dupp"	Abnormal diastole	Incomplete closure of the valves; blood heard regurgitating backward
Friction sound	Abnormal	Inflammation of the heart's pericardial lining; pericarditis

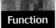
Table 20-3 Peak Expiratory Flow Rate Grading

Color	Zone	Meaning
Green	80% to 100% of personal best	**All clear.** No asthma symptoms are present. Routine treatment plan can be followed. For patients who use medications on a daily basis, consistent measurements in the green zone may allow them to reduce their medications under their physician's guidance.
Yellow	50% to 80% of personal best	**Caution:** An acute attack may be present. Temporary increase in medications may be needed. Consistent readings in this zone may indicate that the condition is not being managed with the current dosage of medications and may need to be increased.
Red	Below 50% of personal best	**Medical alert.** Immediate use of bronchodilators is indicated. If levels do not return immediately to the yellow or green zone after use of the medication, the physician should be notified.

Cardiopulmonary

Box 20–1 Peak Flow Meter (Spirometer)

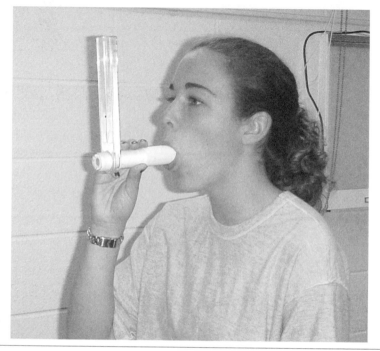

PATIENT POSITION	Standing
POSITION OF EXAMINER	Standing in front of the athlete
EVALUATIVE PROCEDURE	The patient takes as deep a breath as possible. The mouth is placed around the mouthpiece of the peak flow meter. The patient blows as hard and as fast as possible into the device.
POSITIVE TEST	1. Diagnostic: Decreases greater or equal to a 15% decrease in peak expiratory flow rate from pre-exercise to post-exercise. 2. Monitoring: Daily percentage readings of 50 to 80% of personal best or less than 50% of personal best.
IMPLICATIONS	1. Exercise-induced asthma. 2. Asthma attack requiring caution, possibly a temporary increase in bronchodilator dosage or immediate administration of bronchodilators and notification of the treating physician if levels do not return to at least 50% of personal best after medication administration
COMMENT	The patient must be careful not to block the mouthpiece opening with the tongue while performing the test.

21

Skin Conditions

Box 21–1 Common Dermatological Descriptors

Crusts

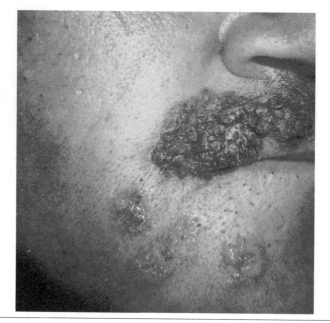

Appearance
Raised layers of dry, crusty skin layers

Color
Yellow-brown
Black

Cause
The collection of serum and inflammatory cells

From Goldsmith, LA, Lazarus, GS, and Tharp, MD: Adult and Pediatric Dermatology: A Color Guide to Diagnosis and Treatment. Philadelphia, FA Davis, 1997.

Box 21-1 Common Dermatological Descriptors (Continued)

Macules

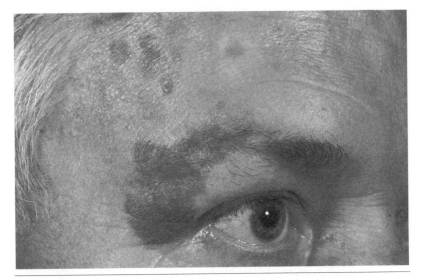

Appearance
Flat

Color
Discolored relative to the surrounding skin

Cause
Pigmentation disorder

Box 21–1 Common Dermatological Descriptors (Continued)

Papules and Plaques

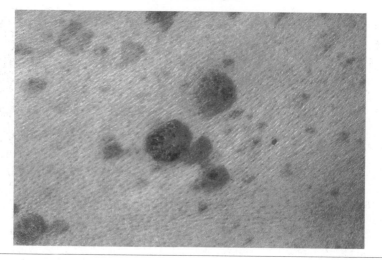

Appearance
Raised
Papules ≤ 1 cm in diameter
Plaques > 1 cm in diameter
Smooth, irregular, or scaly

Color
Brown to black

Cause
Varied

Box 21–1 **Common Dermatological Descriptors** (Continued)

Pustules

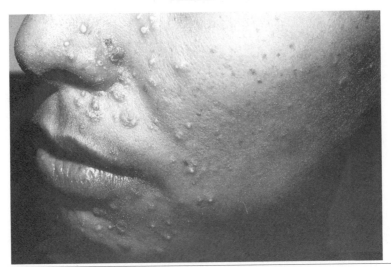

Appearance
Raised
Possible head (pus) formation

Color
Red
Yellow head (pus)

Cause
Infection

Scales

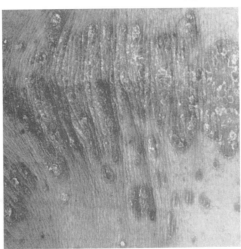

Appearance
Slightly raised
Flaky

Color
Tan

Cause
The proliferation of the normal
shedding of scales from under
the skin

From Goldsmith, LA, Lazarus, GS, and
Tharp, MD: Adult and Pediatric
Dermatology: A Color Guide to
Diagnosis and Treatment. Philadelphia,
FA Davis, 1997..

Box 21–2 Skin Infestations

Scabies

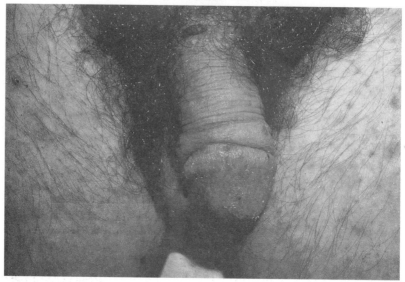

Appearance
Burrows, linear path having a black dot (the scabie mite) at its terminal end
Papules, vesicles, and pustules

Common Sites
Hands
Between the fingers
Wrist and arm
Axilla
Genitals
Inner thighs

Discharge
Pus in the late stages

Sensations
Severe itching

Cause
Infestation by an arachnid mite (*Sarcoptes scabiei*)

Communicable?
Yes
Transmission via direct contact with an infected person; also by sharing clothing,
bedding, and so on (rare)

Treatment
Use Permethrin 5% cream (or similar).
Keep fingernails short to prevent infestation under the nails.
Change bedding regularly.
Keep clothes separated and wash at a high temperature.

From Goldsmith, LA, Lazarus, GS, and Tharp, MD: Adult and Pediatric Dermatology: A Color Guide to
Diagnosis and Treatment. Philadelphia, FA Davis, 1997.

Box 21–2 Skin Infestations (Continued)

Pediculosis (Lice Infestation)

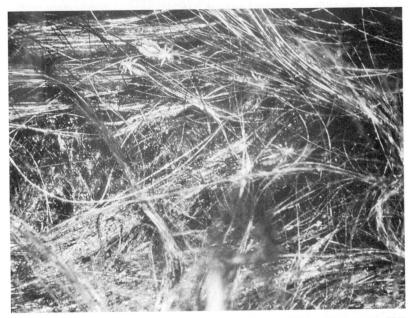

Appearance
Crusting
Scaling
Red eruptions on the skin
The lice or their eggs possibly visible; the eggs resemble dandruff, but remain attached to the hair.

Common Sites
Hair of the head (scalp, beard, eyebrows); infestations common behind the ears
Body hair
Pubic hair (crab lice)

Discharge
Flaking of dry skin

Sensations
Severe itching

Cause
Infestation by lice

Communicable?
Yes
Disease transmission possible by direct contact, sharing of clothing, bedding, hairbrushes, and so on

Treatment
Use over-the-counter shampoos and lotions or prescription medication (e.g., Kwell).
Keep clothes separated and wash at a high temperature.

Skin Conditions

Box 21-3 Common Inflammatory Skin Conditions

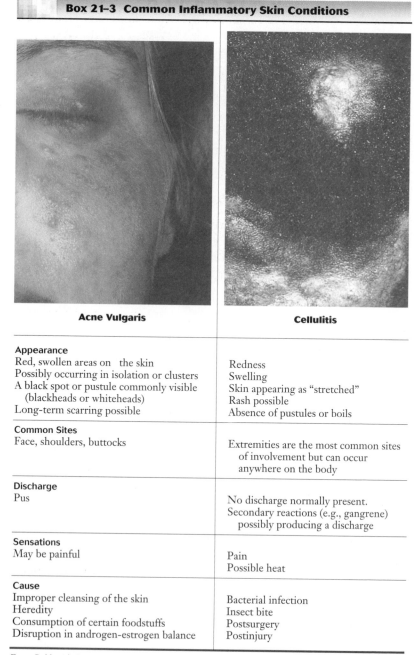

Acne Vulgaris

Cellulitis

Appearance	
Red, swollen areas on the skin	Redness
Possibly occurring in isolation or clusters	Swelling
A black spot or pustule commonly visible (blackheads or whiteheads)	Skin appearing as "stretched"
	Rash possible
Long-term scarring possible	Absence of pustules or boils
Common Sites	
Face, shoulders, buttocks	Extremities are the most common sites of involvement but can occur anywhere on the body
Discharge	
Pus	No discharge normally present. Secondary reactions (e.g., gangrene) possibly producing a discharge
Sensations	
May be painful	Pain
	Possible heat
Cause	
Improper cleansing of the skin	Bacterial infection
Heredity	Insect bite
Consumption of certain foodstuffs	Postsurgery
Disruption in androgen-estrogen balance	Postinjury

From Goldsmith, LA, Lazarus, GS, and Tharp, MD: Adult and Pediatric Dermatology: A Color Guide to Diagnosis and Treatment. Philadelphia, FA Davis, 1997.

Box 21–3 Common Inflammatory Skin Conditions (Continued)

Folliculitis	Contact Dermatitis
Appearance Pustules surrounding hair follicles Growths usually clustered Red rash	Red Inflamed Localized swelling Affected area localized to the skin making contact with the irritant
Common Sites Face and neck Axilla Groin	Anywhere on the body
Discharge Pus discharge from hair follicles possible	Clear seepage possible Crusting frequent
Sensations Itching	Itching Burning
Cause Staph or fungal infection Blockage of the hair follicle Exacerbation with shaving Hot tubs and whirlpool baths as possibly transmitting or causing folliculitis	The skin coming into contact with an irritant (e.g., poison ivy, soap, chemicals)

Box 21–3 Common Inflammatory Skin Conditions (Continued)

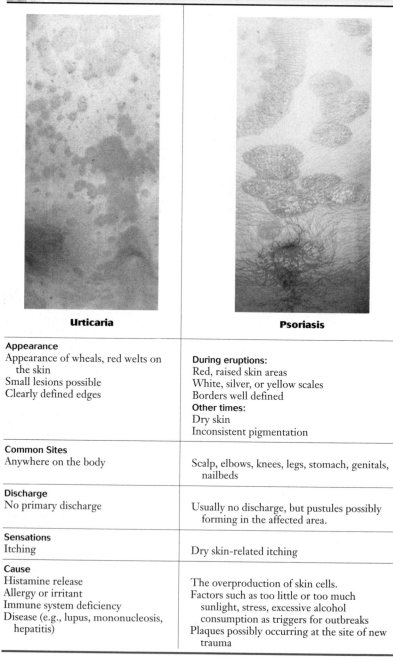

Urticaria	Psoriasis
Appearance Appearance of wheals, red welts on the skin Small lesions possible Clearly defined edges	**During eruptions:** Red, raised skin areas White, silver, or yellow scales Borders well defined **Other times:** Dry skin Inconsistent pigmentation
Common Sites Anywhere on the body	Scalp, elbows, knees, legs, stomach, genitals, nailbeds
Discharge No primary discharge	Usually no discharge, but pustules possibly forming in the affected area.
Sensations Itching	Dry skin-related itching
Cause Histamine release Allergy or irritant Immune system deficiency Disease (e.g., lupus, mononucleosis, hepatitis)	The overproduction of skin cells. Factors such as too little or too much sunlight, stress, excessive alcohol consumption as triggers for outbreaks Plaques possibly occurring at the site of new trauma

Genital Warts

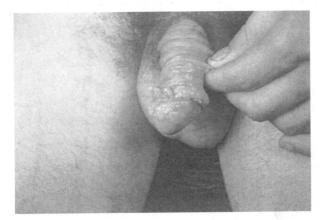

Figure 21–1 Genital warts of the penis.
Courtesy of Schwarz Pharma.

Molluscum Contagiosum

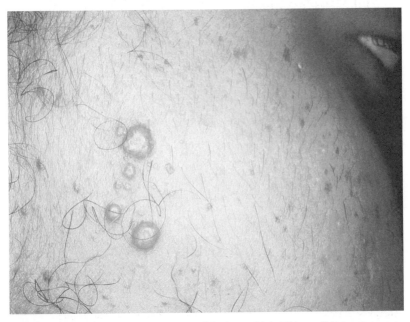

Figure 21–2 Molluscum contagiosum of the inner thigh. This condition may resemble genital warts.
From Goldsmith, LA, Lazarus, GS, and Tharp, MD: Adult and Pediatric Dermatology: A Color Guide to Diagnosis and Treatment. Philadelphia, FA Davis, 1997.

Syphilis

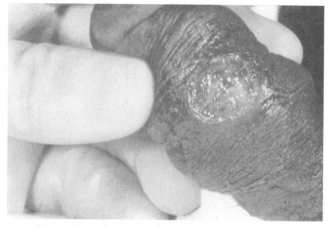

Figure 21–3 Primary syphilitic chancre of the penis.
From Goldsmith, LA, Lazarus, GS, and Tharp, MD: Adult and Pediatric Dermatology: A Color Guide to Diagnosis and Treatment. Philadelphia, FA Davis, 1997.

Herpes Zoster

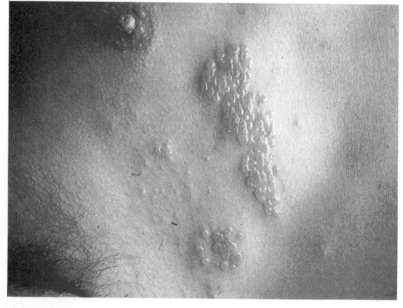

Figure 21–4 Herpes zoster of the chest.
From Goldsmith, LA, Lazarus, GS, and Tharp, MD: Adult and Pediatric Dermatology: A Color Guide to Diagnosis and Treatment. Philadelphia, FA Davis, 1997.

Herpes Simplex

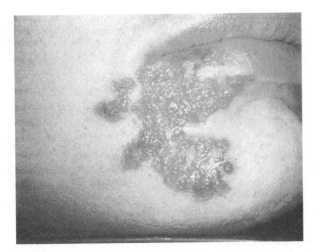

Figure 21–5 Herpes simplex 1 forming the characteristic "cold sore."
Courtesy of Dermick Laboratories, Inc. All rights reserved.

Nodular Melanoma

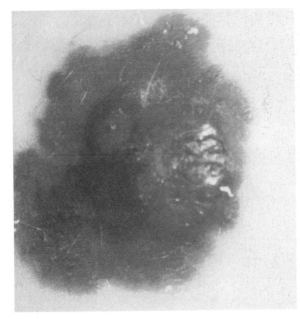

Figure 21–6 Nodular melanoma.
From Goldsmith, LA, Lazarus, GS, and Tharp, MD: Adult and Pediatric Dermatology:
A Color Guide to Diagnosis and Treatment. Philadelphia, FA Davis, 1997.

Leukoplakia

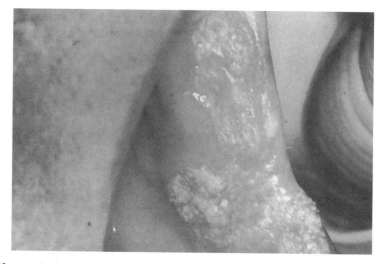

Figure 21–7 Leukoplakia of the tongue.
From Goldsmith, LA, Lazarus, GS, and Tharp, MD: Adult and Pediatric Dermatology: A Color Guide to Diagnosis and Treatment. Philadelphia, FA Davis, 1997.

Cystic Acne

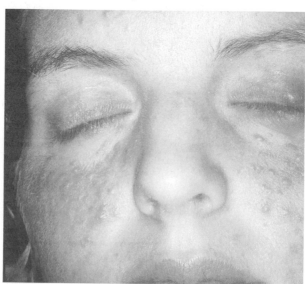

Figure 21–8 Cystic acne of the trunk. This form of acne may leave permanent scarring.
From Goldsmith, LA, Lazarus, GS, and Tharp, MD: Adult and Pediatric Dermatology: A Color Guide to Diagnosis and Treatment. Philadelphia, FA Davis, 1997.

Stasis Dermatitis

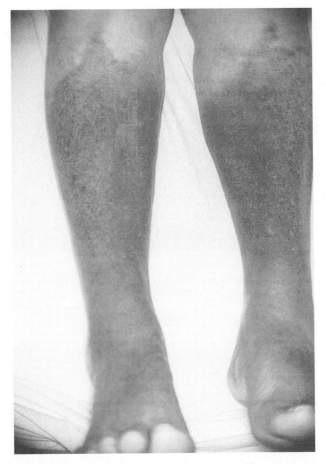

Figure 21–9 Stasis dermatitis of the medial ankle.
From Goldsmith, LA, Lazarus, GS, and Tharp, MD: Adult and Pediatric Dermatology: A Color Guide to Diagnosis and Treatment. Philadelphia, FA Davis, 1997.

Eczema

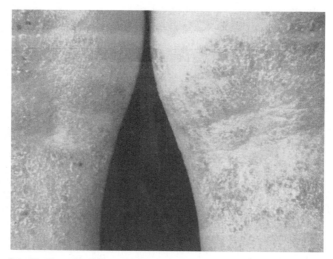

Figure 21–10 Eczema of the posterior legs.
Courtesy of Novartis. All rights reserved.

Impetigo

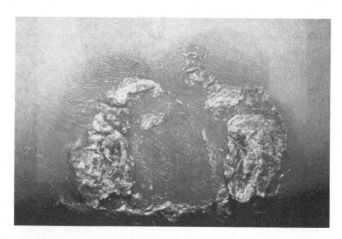

Figure 21–11 Impetigo, a contagious skin condition caused by bacteria.
From Goldsmith, LA, Lazarus, GS, and Tharp, MD: Adult and Pediatric Dermatology: A Color Guide to Diagnosis and Treatment. Philadelphia, FA Davis, 1997.

Ringworm

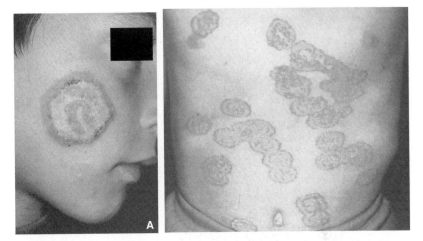

Figure 21–12 Ringworm of the face **(A)** and chest (tinea corporis) **(B)**.
Courtesy of Owen Laboratories.

Tinea Versicolor

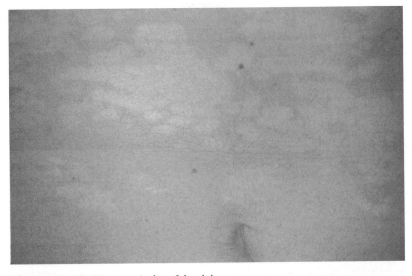

Figure 21–13 Tinea versicolor of the abdomen.
From Goldsmith, LA, Lazarus, GS, and Tharp, MD: Adult and Pediatric Dermatology:
A Color Guide to Diagnosis and Treatment. Philadelphia, FA Davis, 1997.

Warts

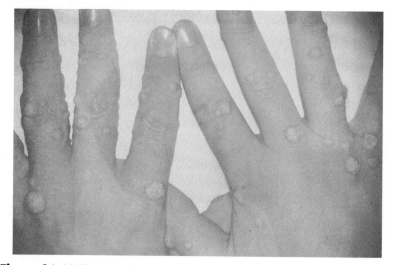

Figure 21–14 Verruca vulgaris (warts) of the hand.
From Goldsmith, LA, Lazarus, GS, and Tharp, MD: Adult and Pediatric Dermatology: A Color Guide to Diagnosis and Treatment. Philadelphia, FA Davis, 1997.

Carbuncle

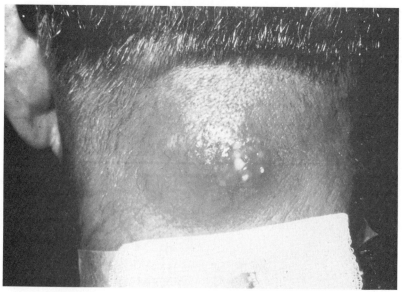

Figure 21–15 Carbuncle of the posterior neck.
From Goldsmith, LA, Lazarus, GS, and Tharp, MD: Adult and Pediatric Dermatology: A Color Guide to Diagnosis and Treatment. Philadelphia, FA Davis, 1997.

Appendix A

Reflex Testing

- **Grade 0:** No reflex elicited
- **Grade 1:** Reflex elicited with reinforcement (hyporeflexia)
- **Grade 2:** Normal reflex
- **Grade 3:** Hyperresponsive reflex

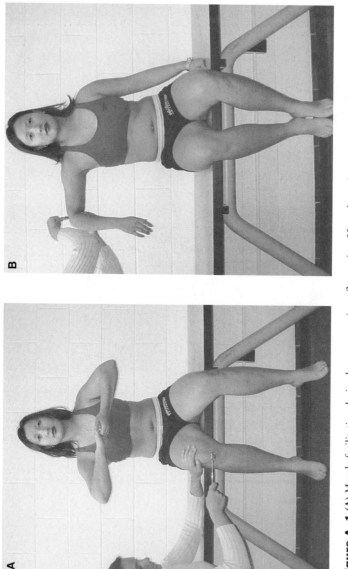

Figure A–1 (A) Muscle facilitation during lower extremity reflex testing. Have the patient attempt to pull the hands apart as shown. **(B)** Muscle facilitation during upper extremity reflex testing. The patient presses the medial aspect of the feet against each other.

Box A–1   C5 Nerve Root Reflex

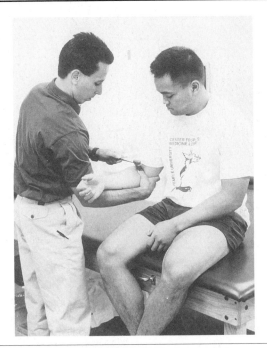

MUSCLE	Biceps brachii
PATIENT POSITION	Seated
POSITION OF EXAMINER	Standing to the side of the patient, cradling the forearm with the thumb placed over the tendon
EVALUATIVE PROCEDURE	The thumb is tapped with the reflex hammer.

Box A-2 C6 Nerve Root Reflex

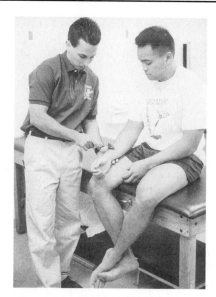

MUSCLE	Brachioradialis
PATIENT POSITION	Seated
POSITION OF EXAMINER	Cradling the patient's arm
EVALUATIVE PROCEDURE	The distal portion of the brachioradialis tendon is tapped with the reflex hammer. The proximal tendon may also be used.

Box A-3 C7 Nerve Root Reflex

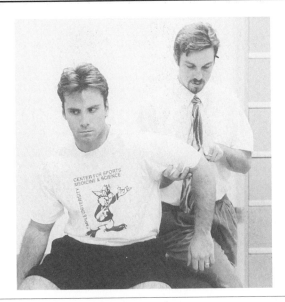

MUSCLE	Triceps brachii
PATIENT POSITION	Seated
POSITION OF EXAMINER	Supporting the athlete's shoulder abducted to 90° and the elbow flexed to 90°
EVALUATIVE PROCEDURE	The distal triceps brachii tendon is tapped with the reflex hammer.

Box A–4 L4 Nerve Root Reflex

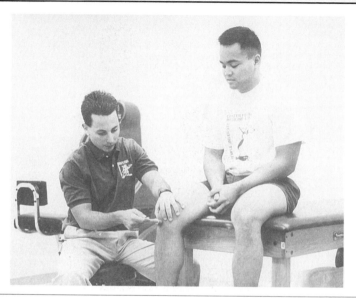

MUSCLE	Patellar tendon (quadriceps femoris)
PATIENT POSITION	Sitting with the knees flexed over the end of the table
POSITION OF EXAMINER	Standing or seated to the side of the athlete
EVALUATIVE PROCEDURE	The patellar tendon is tapped with the reflex hammer.

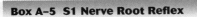

Box A-5   S1 Nerve Root Reflex

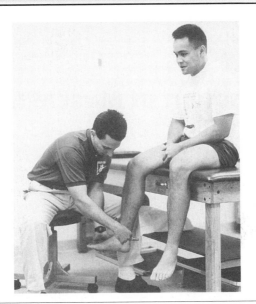

MUSCLE	Achilles tendon (triceps surae muscle group)
PATIENT POSITION	Sitting with the knees flexed over the edge of the table
POSITION OF EXAMINER	Seated in front of the athlete, supporting the foot in its neutral position
EVALUATIVE PROCEDURE	The Achilles tendon is tapped with a reflex hammer.

Appendix A

Appendix B

Assessment of Muscle Length

Box B-1 Muscle Length Assessment for the Gastrocnemius

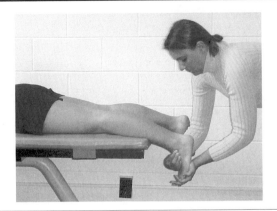

PATIENT POSITION	Prone with the foot off the edge of the table with the knee extended
POSITION OF EXAMINER	One hand palpating the subtalar joint The other hand grasping the foot
EVALUATIVE PROCEDURE	While maintaining the subtalar joint in the neutral position, the foot is taken into dorsiflexion.
POSITIVE TEST	Less than 10° of dorsiflexion for tightness may affect normal walking gait; less than 15° of dorsiflexion may affect normal running gait.
IMPLICATIONS	Tightness of the gastrocnemius can create overuse pathology at the foot, ankle, and knee.
POSSIBLE PATHOLOGIES	Plantar fasciitis, Sever's disease, Achilles tendinitis, calcaneal bursitis, patellofemoral pathology.

Appendix B

Box B–2 Muscle Length Assessment for the Soleus

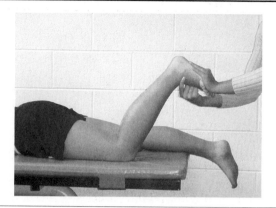

PATIENT POSITION	Prone with the foot off the edge of the table and the knee flexed at least 60°
POSITION OF EXAMINER	One hand palpating the subtalar joint The other hand grasping the foot
EVALUATIVE PROCEDURE	While maintaining the subtalar joint in the neutral position, the foot is taken into dorsiflexion.
POSITIVE TEST	Less than 10° of dorsiflexion for tightness may affect normal walking gait; less than 15° of dorsiflexion may affect normal running gait.
IMPLICATIONS	Tightness of the soleus can create overuse pathology at the foot, ankle, and knee.
POSSIBLE PATHOLOGIES	Plantar fasciitis, Sever's disease, Achilles tendinitis, calcaneal bursitis, patellofemoral pathology

Box B–3 Muscle Length Assessment for the Hamstring Group

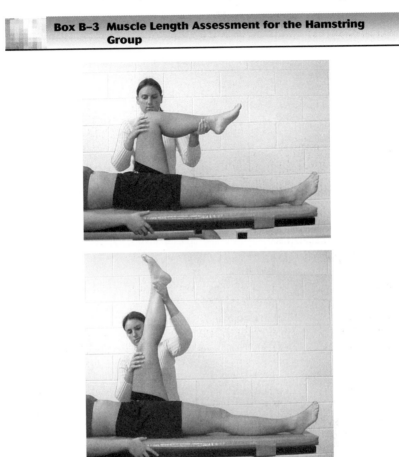

PATIENT POSITION	Supine
POSITION OF EXAMINER	Standing at the side of the patient; the leg being assessed is placed in 90° of hip flexion and 90° of knee flexion (90/90 position)
EVALUATIVE PROCEDURE	The upper leg is stabilized in 90° of hip flexion and the lower leg is extended at the knee.
POSITIVE TEST	Greater than 20° of full knee extension. In patients participating in athletic activities, degrees less than 20° of full knee extension may still be considered as a positive test.
IMPLICATIONS	Tightness of the hamstrings may affect the knee, thigh, hip, and spine.
POSSIBLE PATHOLOGIES	Muscle strains, patellofemoral dysfunction, ischial tuberosity tendinitis, low back pain

Box B-4 Muscle Length Assessment of the Rectus Femoris

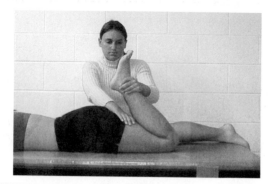

PATIENT POSITION	Prone
POSITION OF EXAMINER	At the side of the patient
EVALUATIVE PROCEDURE	The knee is flexed.
POSITIVE TEST	Less motion than available with ROM testing of the knee in the supine position or 10° or greater difference as compared with the nonaffected side
IMPLICATIONS	Tightness of the quadriceps may affect the knee, thigh, hip, and spine.
POSSIBLE PATHOLOGIES	Muscle strains, patellofemoral dysfunction, hip pain, low back pain

ROM = range of motion.

Box B-5 Muscle Length Assessment of the Shoulder Adductors

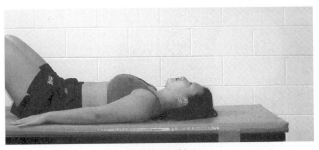

Starting Position

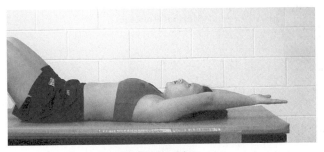

Ending Position

PATIENT POSITION	In the hook-lying position with the arms at the side
POSITION OF EXAMINER	At the side of the patient
EVALUATIVE PROCEDURE	The patient flexes the shoulders above the head and attempts to place the arms on the table.
POSITIVE TEST	The patient cannot flex the arms above the head or the lumbar spine lifts off the table.
IMPLICATIONS	Shortness of the latissimus dorsi and teres major muscles

Appendix B

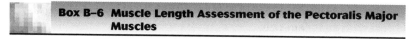

Box B–6 Muscle Length Assessment of the Pectoralis Major Muscles

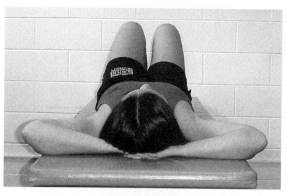

Normal Findings

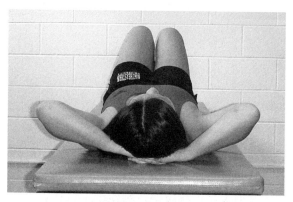

Positive Findings

PATIENT POSITION	In the hook-lying position with the arms abducted, externally rotated, with the elbows flexed and the hands locked behind the head
POSITION OF EXAMINER	At the head of the patient
EVALUATIVE PROCEDURE	The patient attempts to position the elbows flat on the table.
POSITIVE TEST	The elbows do not rest on the table. To establish an objective baseline, measure (in centimeters) the distance from the posterior aspect of the acromion process to the tabletop.
IMPLICATIONS	Tight pectoralis major muscles may create rounded shoulders and subsequent forward head posture.

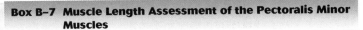

Box B-7 Muscle Length Assessment of the Pectoralis Minor Muscles

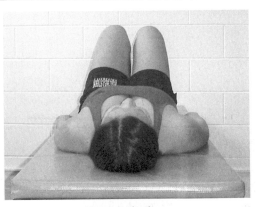

Normal Findings

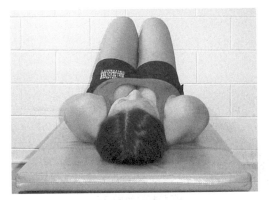

Positive Findings

PATIENT POSITION	Supine with the arms at the side
POSITION OF EXAMINER	At the head of the patient
EVALUATIVE PROCEDURE	Observe the position of the shoulders in reference to the table.
POSITIVE TEST	The posterior shoulder does not rest on the table. To establish an objective baseline, measure (in centimeters) the distance from the posterior aspect of the acromion process to the tabletop.
IMPLICATIONS	Tight pectoralis minor muscles may create rounded shoulders and subsequent forward head posture.

Appendix C

Functional Testing of the Lower Extremity

Box C–1   Single Leg Hop for Distance

Distance

PATIENT POSITION	Standing on one leg
POSITION OF EXAMINER	At the side of the patient
EVALUATIVE PROCEDURE	The patient hops as far as possible, taking off and landing on the same leg. The first set is performed using the uninvolved leg. The second set is performed using the involved leg.
POSITIVE TEST	The distance hopped on the involved leg is less than 85% of the uninvolved leg.

Box C-2 Single Leg Triple Hop for Distance

| | Distance | |

PATIENT POSITION	Standing on one leg
POSITION OF EXAMINER	At the side of the patient
EVALUATIVE PROCEDURE	The patient hops 3 times as far as possible, taking off and landing on the same leg every time. The first set is performed using the uninvolved leg. The second set is performed using the involved leg.
POSITIVE TEST	The distance hopped on the involved leg is less than 85% of the uninvolved leg.

Box C–3 Single Leg Hop for Time

Time required to travel 18 feet

PATIENT POSITION	Standing on one leg
POSITION OF EXAMINER	At the side of the patient
EVALUATIVE PROCEDURE	The patient hops over a distance of 18 ft, taking off and landing on the same leg each time. The first set is performed using the uninvolved leg. The second set is performed using the involved leg.
POSITIVE TEST	The time it takes the patient to hop the distance on the uninvolved leg is less than 85% of the involved leg.

Box C–4　Cross-Over Hop for Distance

Distance

PATIENT POSITION	Standing on one leg
POSITION OF EXAMINER	At the side of the patient
EVALUATIVE PROCEDURE	The patient hops 3 times as far as possible across a line on the floor, taking off and landing on the same leg. The first set is performed using the uninvolved leg. The second set is performed using the involved leg.
POSITIVE TEST	The distance hopped on the involved leg is less than 85% of the uninvolved leg.

Index

Note: Page numbers followed by b indicate boxed material; page numbers followed by f indicate figures; page numbers followed by t indicate tables.

A

Abdomen, 223–233
 percussion of, 230b
Abrasion(s), corneal, fluorescent dye test for, 334b–335b
Achilles tendon rupture, Thompson test for, 90b
ACL. *See* Anterior cruciate ligament (ACL)
Acne, cystic, 384f
Acromiclavicular compression test, 255b
Acromiclavicular traction test, 254b
Active compression test, 268b–269b
Activities of daily living, spinal pain exhibited during, ramifications of, 175t
Acute vulgaris, 378b, 378f
Adson's test, for thoracic outlet syndrome, 270b
Allen test, for thoracic outlet syndrome, 271b
ALRI test, 118b
Amnesia
 anterograde, determination of, 345b
 retrograde, determination of, 344b
Ankle, 72–92
 capsular patterns of, 80t
 goniometry of, 79b
 injuries of
  history of, 74t–75t
  mechanism of, 75t
  tissue damage due to, 75t
 ligamentous stability of, tests for, 84b–87b
 neurologic tests of, 92, 92f
 palpation of, 76–78, 76f–78f
 range of motion of, resisted, 82b–83b
 range-of-motion testing of, 79–83, 79b, 80f, 80t, 81f, 82b, 83b
Anterior cruciate ligament (ACL), laxity of
 anterior drawer test for, 106b
 Lachman's test for, 107b
Anterior drawer test, 84b
 for ACL laxity, 106b
Anterior glenohumeral laxity
 apprehension test for, 253b
 relocation test for, 256b
Anterograde amnesia, determination of, 345b
Anterolateral instability, of knee, lateral pivot shift test for, 117b

Anterolateral rotatory instability, of knee, flexion-reduction drawer test for, 119b
Ape hand, 295b, 295f
Apley's compression and distraction tests, for meniscal lesions, 124b
Apley's scratch tests, 244b–245b
Apprehension test
 for anterior glenohumeral laxity, 253b
 posterior, for glenohumeral laxity, 257b
 for subluxating/dislocating patella, 142b
Arm, upper, 234–273. *See also under* Shoulder
 inspection of, 236f
 ligamentous tests of, 250b–251b
 neurologic testing of, 273f
 palpation of, 237–239, 237f, 238f
 range-of-motion testing of, 240–249, 240b–241b, 242t, 243f, 244b–249b
Arthritis, evaluative findings in, 23t
Articular fractures, 25b
Athletic competitions, in hot environments, modifications of, 364t

B

Babinski test, for upper motor neuron lesions, 221b
Balance error scoring system (BESS), after head and neck injuries, 352b–353b
Beevor's sign, for thoracic nerve inhibition, 186b
Biceps brachii pathology, Ludington's test for, 267b
Biceps brachii tendinitis, long head of, Speed's test for, 266b
Biceps tendon, subluxation of, Yergason's test for, 264b–265b
Bishop's deformity, 296b, 296f
Blood pressure, assessment of, 232b
Blowout fracture, 329f
Body types, classications of, 28b
Bony injuries, evaluative findings in, 24t–25t, 25b–27b
 exostosis, 24t
 stress fractures, 24t–25t
Boutonnière deformity, 300b, 300f
Brachial plexus traction test, 214b